THE **5 PILLARS** OF
RUNES

FOUNDATION   LAYOUTS AND SPREADS   RUNIC SCRIPTS   CASTING   READING

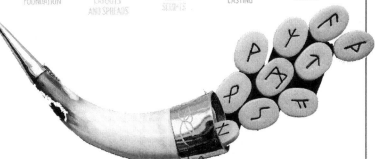

97 TECHNIQUES & INSIGHTS
to Connect to Your Higher Self Through the Magic and Rituals of Runelore. Tap Into Your Intuition by Harnessing the Power and Wisdom of Runic Symbols

INGRID CLARKE

© Copyright 2023 - All rights reserved.

The content contained within this book may not be reproduced, duplicated, or transmitted without direct written permission from the author or the publisher.

Under no circumstances will any blame or legal responsibility be held against the publisher, or author, for any damages, reparation, or monetary loss due to the information contained within this book, either directly or indirectly.

Legal Notice:

This book is copyright protected. It is only for personal use. You cannot amend, distribute, sell, use, quote, or paraphrase any part, or the content within this book, without the author's or publisher's consent.

Disclaimer Notice:

Please note that the information contained within this document is for educational and entertainment purposes only. All effort has been executed to present accurate, up-to-date, reliable, and complete information. No warranties of any kind are declared or implied. Readers acknowledge that the author does not render legal, financial, medical, or professional advice. The content within this book has been derived from various sources. Please consult a licensed professional before attempting any techniques outlined in this book.

By reading this document, the reader agrees that under no circumstances is the author responsible for any direct or indirect losses incurred as a result of the use of the information contained within this document, including, but not limited to, errors, omissions, or inaccuracies.

Table of Contents

Introduction 5

Pillar 1: Foundation... 9

Chapter 1: Foundation 11
    Defining Runes 11
    Using the Runes 18

Pillar 2: Runic Scripts 23

Chapter 2: Different Runic Scripts 25
    Early Germanic 25
    Anglo-Saxon 27
    Nordic 28
    Medieval 30

Chapter 3: Elder Futhark 33
    The Aetts of the Elder Futhark 33

Chapter 4: Younger Futhark 51
    History of the Younger Futhark 52
    The Runes of the Younger Futhark 53

Chapter 5: Anglo-Saxon Futhorc 67
    History of the Anglo-Saxon Futhorc 68
    The Runes of the Futhorc 69

Pillar 3: Casting 95

Chapter 6: What You Need to Know About Rune Casting .. 97
    History of Rune Casting 98
    How to Cast Runes 99
    Tools of the Trade 105

Pillar 4: Layouts and Spreads 109

Chapter 7: Layouts and Spreads List 111
    Runic Layouts and Spreads 112

Pillar 5: Reading 121

Chapter 8: Interpreting Runes 123
    Casting and Interpreting Runes 124

Conclusion 137

References 139

Introduction

Are you struggling to make sense of a meaningful life event? Do you feel like the universe is trying to tell you something, but you cannot understand what it is saying? Runes could be the answer. These ancient symbols hold the power of the cosmos and offer insights, protection, and divine knowledge that can unlock the answers to some of life's most difficult questions. Unlike many forms of divination, rune reading has been around for centuries and was used by our ancestors to seek guidance. They believe runes have a unique ability to tap into unseen forces and energies that provide a deeper understanding of ourselves and our place in the world. With their help, you can gain clarity in any situation, find direction when lost, and discover a new purpose in life.

Likewise, runes can give us a glimpse into deeper truths hidden from our everyday view. By understanding how to use and solve them, you can learn how to read unseen threads of fate and even rewrite your destiny. This book provides a comprehensive guide on runecraft, exploring the five pillars of runology: rune scripts, spreads and layouts, interpretation based on questions asked, and more. As you journey through this initiatory process into the world of runology, you will gain an insightful new lens through which to view life's complexities. The information in this book will give you a firm footing in recognizing when life calls for you to invoke the wisdom of runes, unlocking their language and your potential.

Everyone faces trials and tribulations that can be hard to bear. But true strength lies in those who strive to overcome these difficulties and learn more about themselves and our world. Our modern society is saturated with technology, making it easy to become disconnected from our environment. Also, it leads us to lose not only sight of nature but also the spiritual power within ourselves. Engaging with our natural surroundings can reconnect with life's mysteries and foster greater well-being.

Having endured burnout in the past and coming from a Scandinavian family with Pagan roots, I have dedicated my life to exploring different healing practices. I have gained incredible insight into metaphysical practices and occult traditions from all over the world. Likewise, I feel a unique connection to the runes, those magnificent cosmic symbols so beloved by my ancestors. As an empath, it is my role to pass on the extensive knowledge and wisdom I have acquired through my long years of research on bringing relief to those who need it. Furthering this quest is my deep appreciation for herbalism, crystal healing, astrology, and spiritual philosophies.

This book delves deep into the study of runes, providing insightful knowledge into where they come from and how to use them. You will find 97 techniques, tips, and strategies on how to explore the transformative world of runecraft, offering a journey of self-discovery and spiritual enlightenment, peppered throughout the entire book. It's intentionally designed this way to serve as your guide along each step of the process.

Uncover the history of runes, including the Elder Futhark and Younger Futhark as well as the Anglo-Saxon futhorc. That said, you will gain a thorough understanding of these ancient symbols. Yet, not only will this book educate readers in casting and interpreting runes based on whatever question is asked or layout is chosen. As such, it also offers detailed knowledge about various spreads and layouts. Hence, this book gives insight into this powerful yet simple approach to uncovering the truth.

Unraveling the secrets of our fate can be daunting, especially when life's obstacles seem to stand in our way. But with the use of runes, we can gain insight into our future and uncover the mysteries that are hidden from us. Through my research and publishing of the techniques I share in this book, I have better understood myself and aligned with a path forward. Utilizing these special symbols has allowed me to strengthen my awareness. Likewise, I have become more prepared to decipher life's cosmic puzzles.

The end goal of this book is to help you on a journey of spiritual enlightenment and awakening. Also, it will guide you in tapping into your intuition, understanding your motivation, building self-confidence, and making decisions that will lead you to a better tomorrow. Embark on a voyage of self-discovery by unlocking the runes' secrets and uncovering the divine power within us all. Through rune wisdom and reading, you will be given an insight into life's complexities that can open your eyes to new perspectives. Furthermore, this knowledge can provide practical advice on how to apply them in real-life situations. Plus, guide you toward attaining personal growth and clarity. Let us begin this fantastic journey.

Pillar 1
Foundation

Crafting a solid foundation is an essential part of any learning journey. An apt analogy to this process is building a house. The structure must be sound before anything else can be constructed. In this chapter, we will ensure that your fundamental understanding is adequately cemented in place. This foundational knowledge will act as the base upon which more complex topics can be developed, helping to ensure that you build your understanding logically and systematically. Additionally, having real-world relevant facts or examples connected to this information can help strengthen your grasp of the subject.

1

What you need to know about Runes

There is much mystery surrounding the origins of the runic symbols. Tales from Norse mythology tell of how Odin, ruler in chief of Asgard and a most revered god among the Norse Pantheon, sacrificed himself on Yggdrasil, the cosmic tree connecting Nine Worlds. Hanging for nine days and nine nights, he was able to unlock the mysteries of the universe symbolized by runes. By definition, runes are inscribed characters or symbols believed to have magical properties. It was through his immense sacrifice that Odin revealed their hidden meaning. Such stories perpetuate the mythos associated with runes, which embed themselves in our collective imaginations as we explore their history and purpose.

Defining Runes

The runes are not just used for divination and magic, but they also carry much historical significance. Used by many Germanic societies from the 1st to 2nd century AD, these runes have been adopted into various languages that use the Latin alphabet. Unlike today's Latin alphabet, each rune is an ideogram representing sounds, objects, or ideas. Thinking about it, they are much like Egyptian hieroglyphs or Ancient Chinese characters. This uniqueness makes them invaluable tools for divination, fortune-telling, and advice-seeking. Furthermore, many medieval scholars believed runes could be used as powerful talismans to protect oneself from misfortunes. All these make runes a fascinating part of history.

Definition

Learning about something new can be an exciting journey, especially regarding runes. As the Merriam-Webster Dictionary outlines, runes have three distinct meanings. As such, these three are the characters used by early Germanic people, mystery and magic, and Old Norse poetry or songs. Moreover, another interpretation of this ancient alphabet is *"secret conversation"* or *" something hidden."* Hence, a concept that carries a certain degree of power. This power is further emphasized with reference to Norse mythology, which tells of an origin story for runes where each letter holds both a sound and a concept. Through this lens, it becomes clear why rune-speaking people believed in the strength of words so strongly that they embedded symbols of power in their letters.

Linguistic History

From ancient Nordic tribes to modern-day esoteric practitioners, runes have been used across time and cultures as a written form of communication. Three of the most renowned alphabets crafted from runes are—

Elder Futhark

The Germanic runic alphabet, also known as Elder Futhark, was an ancient script used by Germanic tribes in Northwest Germany during the Migration Period. Made up of 24 runes, it got its name from its first six letters *(F, U, Þ, A, R, and K)*, which spelled out 'futhark.' An example of one of these tribes was the Goths, who are believed to be among the first to have adopted this writing system. Despite being labeled as *'barbarians,'* they defeated the Roman empire. Also, they gained recognition for their powerful alphabetic system that held many esoteric meanings. In addition, some early Christian missionaries used these runes as a tool to spread their message, providing further evidence of their importance throughout history.

As we have mentioned before, using runes for magic or divination purposes predates the creation of the alphabet itself. During the time the Elder Futhark was created, writing was considered to be a tool for magic. There were only a select few in each tribe who had the skill to write and read these magical signs known as runes. Spells were cast using the runes, fortunes told, and secret messages. The Elder Futhark writing system itself is considered to have been a *"secret"* language of symbols. Through its hidden lore, the power of the gods could be brought into the physical world, and the will of the inscriber made manifest.

Anglo-Saxon Futhorc

The second prominent runic alphabet used by the Anglo-Saxons was the 'Futhorc,' derived from earlier Germanic runes. It was brought to Britain when three powerful Germanic tribes, the Angles, Saxons, and Jutes, invaded in the 5th century AD. Each tribe had its language. As such, Old English for the Angles, Old Saxon for the Saxons, and Old Jute for the Jutes were written using Futhorc. After conquering Britain, Anglo-Saxons brought their culture and traditions to their new lands. They also brought Norse mythology and beliefs, which blended into local Celtic folklore. Subsequently, it gave rise to a unique culture that can still be seen today in British customs and traditions.

For half a millennium, the Anglo-Saxons developed their version of the popular Germanic writing system known as runes. Adapting the Elder Futhark alphabet, they utilized new symbols and amassed 33 characters. Then, nine more than its parent and 17 more than the Younger Futhark. In doing so, they could transpose their language, Old English, onto stone and parchment for future generations to study. This adaptation of an ancient script is a testament to the Anglo-Saxon's dedication to preserving their culture and history.

Younger Futhark

The Younger Futhark, or Scandinavian Runes, was used by the Vikings from 793 to 1066 A.D. as a form of communication and record-keeping. This writing system had only 16 runes compared to the 24 that its predecessor, the Elder Futhark, had. The main reason for simplifying the runic alphabet is to increase literacy levels among the Germanic tribe. Plus, there is a growing need for writing down more complex information. As a result, it has become an essential part of Viking history and culture, with many rune stones still standing today.

Besides, the Elder Futhark was an ancient writing system used mainly by the elite for divination or other magical purposes. Meanwhile, Younger Futhark was widely used and adopted by people of all social classes across Scandinavia. Consequently, it was simplified to make carving messages on stones, making it a valuable communication tool. Even though the 350 existing inscriptions of Elder Futhark are scarce compared to the more than 3000 runestones written in Younger Futhark, they cover a broad spectrum. As such, they include prophecies, everyday conversations, and even humorous remarks. Evidently, its success lies in its ability to enable ordinary people to leave behind a tangible trace of their culture, ideas, and thoughts.

Medieval Runes

Emerging from the Younger Futhark of the 13th century, Medieval Runes, or Futhork, consisted of 27 characters and were used across Scandinavia in the Middle Ages. This script also served as the basis for the highly popular runology of the 16th century, with many runes modified or taken directly from existing symbols in the Younger Futhark. Tracing back further, these runes originated from the Older Futhark. While the meanings of these runes stayed largely unaltered, their sound representation and physical shape varied considerably between different alphabets. To highlight this development even more, it is believed that some runes were explicitly developed to represent new sounds that arose during this period.

Latin Writing Invades

In the late 11th century, the Latin alphabet became a competitor to the Futhork in Scandinavia. However, since it was still expensive to write with a quill and ink on parchment, essential for Latin writing, the clergy mainly used it. Meanwhile, the Old Norse language continued to be written down using runes carved on wood, stone, or other hard surfaces using sharp objects. Likewise, Latin prayers and many Medieval church objects display rune engravings. These include medieval runes engraved on church bells, baptismal fonts, and relic containers carved on church doors, walls, and front porches.

During the 13th century, Latin writing began supplanting runes and was used to write down medieval Scandinavian laws. This transition quickly led to Latin becoming the dominant writing system among politicians and clergypersons. Although the public transitioned from using runes to Latin letters, some still maintained the usage of runes for various esoteric purposes such as divination, magic, and secret messages. The study of runology eventually rose after rune scholars in the 16th century started studying their history and using it academically. Additionally, several manuscripts documenting Nordic mysteries and spells were composed during this period, testifying how runes were kept alive in Nordic culture even when Latin had become popularized.

The Birth of Runology

Runology is an ancient and powerful field of study that traces back to Johannes Bureus in the 16th century. He was the royal librarian for the King of Sweden and believed that the runes had a practical use and held mystical and holy properties. This spiritual belief has been strengthened recently due to archaeological evidence, such as rare runestones, linking it to prosperity, longevity, and protection. Bureus' larger contribution to Swedish culture included being a tutor and advisor to King Gustavus Adolphus. Likewise, he was considered the *"father of Swedish grammar."* As such, his work can be seen throughout Scandinavian culture today. This commitment to preserving Old Norse culture earned him recognition as a proponent of Gothicism with solid ties to the Geats. Besides, he claimed they were direct descendants of those who conquered the Roman Empire. Likewise, he believed that runes, the Old Norse tribe's writing system, were not just letters like those in Latin. Yet, they were something extraordinary and even sacred.

Mythological Origins

I know I hung on that windswept tree,
Swung there for nine long nights,
Wounded by my own blade,
Bloodied for Odin,
Myself an offering to myself:
Bound to the tree
That no man knows

Whither the roots of it run.

None gave me bread,
None gave me drink.
Down to the deepest depths, I peered.
Until I spied the Runes.
With a roaring cry, I seized them up,
Then dizzy and fainting, I fell.

Well-being, I won.
And wisdom too.
From a word to a word
I was led to a word,
From a deed to another deed.
(Poetic Edda, ca.1200 AD, The Speech of the High One)

The poem above tells the tale of Odin All-father, the chief of Norse mythology. He acquired knowledge of runes by performing a ritualistic sacrifice, suspending himself from Yggdrasil for nine nights and days. Known as a source of great wisdom, Urd's Well lies directly below Yggdrasil's branches, where Odin saw symbols of the universe encoded within it. This divine insight likely made him the most powerful god among Germanic tribes. To commemorate his achievement, *Wednesday, or "Woden's Day,"* is still named after him. Moreover, many attribute Odin with abilities such as wisdom, knowledge, sorcery, and poetry, all governed by the runic alphabet.

Meanwhile, stories involving Odin are often associated with his deepened knowledge of the universe's mysteries. He famously drank from the Mead of Poetry, an enchanted elixir that granted him the power to become a *'skald'* or scholar. Its ability allowed him to remember and recite any information learned and to solve any problem he set his mind to. As a result, he was revered as the great magician and All-father of the Norse Pantheon.

With this knowledge and power, Odin was also seen as the perfect being to understand runes and teach others how to read them.

The Germanic tribes did not believe these symbols had been invented or created. Instead, they saw them as pre-existing forces of the cosmos which Odin imparted upon certain people, known as runemasters. As such, this way allows them to interpret their powerful meanings for divination purposes or engrave them for protection and magic spells. Additionally, these runes were considered a source of wisdom that could connect one with spiritual guidance or ancestral knowledge.

Using the Runes

Now that we know more about their linguistic history and mythological origins, it is time to explore the uses of runes. Not only were they used as a writing system, but they also served as a tool for magic or divination. Runes were inscribed in places of importance and even within Christian churches, calling upon the gods for protection and blessing. Furthermore, runes were found engraved on swords, ceremonial and used in battle, carved onto wooden strips, or painted on pebbles or stones for divination. With this new knowledge, runes can be seen as symbols of communication and conduits of spiritual power with various applications in both protective and predictive realms.

The first historical record we have of Germanic peoples using the runes for divine or occult purposes comes from Tacitus, the renowned Roman historian, and politician, who wrote a detailed account of it in his book *Germania 10* (98AD):

> *"They attach the highest importance to taking auspices and casting lots. Their usual procedure with the lot is simple. They cut off a branch from a nut or seed-bearing tree and slice it*

into strips; they mark it with different signs and throw them randomly onto a white cloth. Then the state's priest, if it is an official consultation, or the father of the family, in a private one, offers prayer to the gods and, looking up towards heaven, picks up three strips, one at a time, and, according to which sign they have previously been marked with, makes his interpretation."

Ancient runes have been around for centuries, having been discovered and decoded by multiple civilizations. Odin was believed to be the god of prophecy, who gifted our species with his powerful symbols. As we delve into these symbols and the practice of rune reading, it is essential to remember that they have been used as a form of divination and magic for more than two millennia. This ancient insight can be applied to this day to bring new clarity and understanding into our lives.

Casting and Drawing Runes

Uncovering further knowledge and insights lies at the heart of rune casting. Each rune is a double-edged sword, containing both an *'external'* and *'internal'* meaning. Its main purpose is as a pictogram to tap into cosmic powers for divination. After preparing the space for your runes, place them onto a flat surface to protect them from sliding and bouncing around too much. Once cast, they are interpreted in terms of where they lay relative to the caster and how they are arranged compared to other runes used in that casting session. Learn more about unlocking these mysteries in chapter six of runelore: casting. Commit to learning more about runes and rune casting to get the most out of your readings. Their secrets are waiting for you to uncover.

Another way to practice divination with runes is called 'drawing runes.' This is similar to drawing a card from a tarot deck.

The diviner can lay the runes face-down on a flat surface or pull them out of an opaque bag. In one method, the diviner passes their non-dominant hand over the face-down runes until they feel attracted to one that stands out, then flips it and interprets its meaning. In the second method, three runes are drawn from the bag, one at a time. These individual rune readings are then interpreted as part of a larger reading according to what was asked when starting the divination process. Some believe that which rune is chosen or drawn is determined by the spiritual energies present in their environment at that moment.

Runecraft and Runic Magic

> *"Beer, I bring thee, tree of battle,*
> *Mingled of strength and mighty fame.*
> *Charms it holds and healing signs,*
> *Spells full good, and gladness-runes."*
> **(Burrows, 2007, p.139)**

Runes are sacred symbols in Norse mythology inscribed on stones, wood, and objects to divine the future or call upon supernatural powers. These same runes can be used to cast spells as they were believed to have a connection with the gods. In the poem *Sigrdrífumál*, *Brynhildr* bestows a beer blessed with runes of joy and gladness upon Sigurd. The Poetic Edda is a legendary collection of Old Norse poems thought to have been written between 800-1150 AD. This work of literature is an integral part of Norse folklore and provides an insight into how pre-Christian Scandinavians viewed their world.

Brynhildr then explains the various magical uses of the runes for the following seven stanzas. Here is an overview of the different uses Brynhildr mentions.

- **Victory Runes.** Carved and used on sword hilts to ensure victorious combat.
- **Ale Runes (ølrunar).** Used as a protective charm against being bewitched through ale served by a host's wife.
- **Birth Runes (biargrunar).** Utilized in childbirth to help aid safe delivery.
- **Wave Runes (brimrunar).** Incanted and carved on the stem and rudder of ships for protection from sea dangers.
- **Branch Runes (limrunar).** Scribed onto east-facing trees for healing purposes.
- **Speech Runes (malrunar).** Inscribed to enhance one's rhetoric skills.
- **Thought Runes (hugrunar).** Engraved to sharpen the mind.

Knowledge of rune magic and divination has been around for centuries, tracing its roots back to the Middle Ages. Runes have a rich history with many cultures and languages, containing immense power and potential in their use. With this foundational understanding of runes, you can now begin to explore the possibilities their symbols can bring to your life. In the next chapter, we will dive into Runic Scripts to understand how different languages use these runic alphabets. To make sure you get as much out of runes as possible, it is essential to research their origin before using them. As such, some have been known to have strong ties with ancient Norse mythology. With that in mind, may you soon enjoy the fortuitousness that casting and reading runes can bring.

Pillar 2
Runic Scripts

With our understanding of runology as a foundation, it is time to explore the next pillar: runic scripts. Runes were used for many purposes, including divination and magic, but their primary use was as letters of the alphabet. Ancient runic artifacts, such as rune staffs carved with symbols, provide us with tangible evidence that runes were used to form written language. It is possible to organize your knowledge of runes by viewing them through the lens of the three main runic alphabets: *Elder Futhark, Younger Futhark, and Anglo-Saxon Futhorc.* Understanding these alphabets requires an overview of the runic script, what it is, and how it functions within its given context.

2

Different Runic Scripts

From the 3rd century to the 16th or 17th century, Germanic people in northern Europe, Britain, Scandinavia, and Iceland used runes as a writing system. A late arrival in the history of writing systems, these pictographs are far older than the alphabets they were incorporated into. This chapter will explore the three early runic scripts. As such, it will trace their spread and evolution and delve into the tribes and cultures that harnessed them. Let us step towards mastering runelore as we discover more about their past. Connecting with a mythical past filled with power and depth, runes can bring wisdom and insight to our lives today.

Early Germanic

The Elder Futhark is an ancient runic alphabet combining elements from Proto-Indo-European and indigenous Northern European cultures. It was in use until the 8th century AD, after which other variations of Runic alphabets, like Anglo-Saxon Futhorc, emerged. This script was inscribed on objects ranging from jewelry to weapons, indicating its widespread usage in Northern Europe during this period.

At the time of Elder Futhark's emergence, the world was experiencing a period known as Late Antiquity. New technology, including iron weapons and tools, replaced bronze during this transitional period, marking a dramatic shift in many cultures' practices. This shift set into motion the Migration Period (300–800 AD), where Early Germanic tribes invaded and settled in areas formerly occupied by the Western Roman Empire, an event now affectionately referred to as *"Barbarian Invasions."* The early Germanic tribes brought their writing system, Elder Futhark, with them as they spread through Europe over five centuries.

The Runic Script Heads Abroad

The Migration Period was a time of immense cultural change in Europe, and with it came the spread of the Elder Futhark script. This ancient Germanic alphabet was widely adopted from Germany throughout Scandinavia, western Europe, and even as far east as Poland, Ukraine, and Romania. During this period, the Elder Futhark was a source of stability for new settlers across many nations, providing a common language to trade goods and express ideas. In addition, it also provided an invaluable link to their shared cultural past by connecting pre-Christian Germanic mythology with local Pagan practices throughout Europe.

Scholars trace the beginnings of the Elder Futhark, a runic alphabet that originated in a fusion of Roman and Gothic culture, to an uncertain date between 1 BC and 5 AD. This belief is contested by some who believe that it was first developed as early as 27 BC. The oldest surviving example of this writing system is an ancient runestone in Sweden that dates back to the 5th century AD. Aside from providing insight into their origin, this script has long been used as a form of communication and divination by many cultures worldwide, including Scandinavia, Britain, and Germany.

Moreover, ancient runes serve as a relic of the past and contain much history. One such artifact is the *Spearhead of Kovel*, discovered 30km outside of Kovel, Ukraine, in the early 3rd century. The runes inscribed on it are believed to be *"thither rider"* in Danish translation. This victory rune was not meant as a boast but as an offering to Odin himself. The immense spiritual significance of spears at that time had been deeply embedded in Germanic culture, particularly among the Goths, who treated these weapons with magical reverence. Through these artifacts, we can better understand the rich mythology and beliefs held by our ancestors.

Likewise, from the mysticism and mythology of Early Germanic people, runes have long held special meaning and purpose. During the 7th to 9th centuries AD, the Elder Futhark underwent a transfiguration, resulting in two distinct runic alphabets. This period marked the Viking Age's start, characterized by European exploration and colonization. Plus, it was indicated the time when runes began to be used for political means, personal reflections, and stories of everyday life.

Anglo-Saxon

During the Viking Age, the Norsemen pillaged, plundered, conquered, and colonized much of Europe. In addition to their settlements in the British Isles and Ireland, Greenland, and Normandy, they even reached eastern Europe. One of the most daring Vikings set foot in North America when they landed in Newfoundland, making them the first Europeans to do so. The Norse Peoples also established formidable kingdoms and earldoms across Europe and Britain. As such, it includes York *(Jórvík)* in northern Northumbria and Dublin *(Dyflin)* in Ireland. Along with their culture and traditions, they brought their distinctive runic writing system with them as they spread across northern Europe and the British Isles.

The Celts, originating from the Germanic region, made their way to Britain as early as 500 BC. Yet, there is no surviving evidence of them using runes or any writing system. This may be attributed to their quick conquest and colonization by the Romans, who viewed anyone outside Rome as 'barbarians' rather than preserving their history. During this period, Latin reigned as the predominant writing system of the British Isles. Despite that, its use was limited due to a lack of literacy.

However, during the invasion of Britain in the 5th century AD by the Angles, Saxons, and Jutes, the runes are believed to have been documented in history books. After winning over the Romans, the Anglo-Saxons stayed primarily in England. They also evolved into what is now known as the English race, while Ireland, Scotland, and Wales retained more Celtic influence. The areas controlled by the Anglo-Saxons contained abundant evidence of rune usage.

Nordic

As the Elder Futhark evolved into the Anglo-Saxon Futhorc in Britain, a transformation occurred on the European continent. Coinciding with the Viking Age came the onset of the Younger Futhark. Although these two runic scripts derived from the Elder Futhark, they had some critical differences. The primary distinction is that while extra runes were added to the Futhorc, eight were removed from the Younger Futhark, leaving only 16 characters. This notion of simplification started in the late 7th century and was finalized around the 9th century when Vikings held sway over much of Europe. This period created the shapes and styles we commonly associate with runes today and their most renowned wielders: *The Norsemen or the Vikings.*

Younger Futhark and the Viking Age

The Younger Futhark is believed to have been in use since around 800 AD, and its arrival changed the history of writing as we know it. As it spread rapidly across Scandinavia and Viking Age settlements, these runes were used by kings, warriors, traders, and citizens. As such, they use runes for various reasons when documenting, creating a love letter, or invoking the gods. Subsequently, the rune alphabet was versatile enough to be used for anything a person desired.

Compared to its predecessor, the Elder Futhark, a *"secret"* script solely known and used by the literate elites for religious purposes. Yet, this Younger Futhark opened up literacy and writing to all levels of society. Old Norse continued as mainly a spoken language. However, writing increased drastically due to the introduction of these versatile runes that could do just about anything.

As the Younger Futhark arose, it was divided into two dialects. These two are the Danish long-branch runes and Swedish or Norwegian short-twig runes. The former was used for inscriptions on stone. Meanwhile, the latter was for everyday purposes. Yet, both are private and official carved into the wood. Over time, the short-twig runes evolved into a simpler version of their long-branch counterparts. In the 10th century AD, these further simplified runes took form in a dialect called *"Hälsinge"* or *" staveless runes."* This dialect originated in Hälsingland, Sweden. Also, it was the culmination of a gradual process that began with Elder Futhark giving way to its younger variation. These staveless runes are so named because they typically omit their stave (vertical line), making it easier to write longer texts.

However, attempts to adapt the Younger Futhark runes for everyday use failed, with Latin eventually becoming the preferred writing system throughout Scandinavia as the region became increasingly Christianized. By the 12th century, Latin was overwhelmingly used for writing in Scandinavia, and the runes reverted to their original purpose as a 'secret' script.

Medieval

As the Viking Age neared its close, the invention of dotted runes, known as stung, ushered in the Futhork, or *"Medieval Runes."* This new set of runes added a dot or bar accent marker to simplify the Younger Futhark's issue of one rune representing more than one sound. The various accents distinguished between *'i,' 'e,'* and *'j'* runes depending on whether a dot, bar, or nothing was present.

By the early 13th century, the medieval runic alphabet had been fully formed. This alphabet expanded the 16 characters in the Younger Futhark, eventually reaching 27. Those who carved runes, known as runemasters, often chose to use and modify existing runes rather than make new ones. In this way, many of the runes featured in the Futhark were directly derived from those in the Elder Futhark. Although there may be subtle differences between versions of these ancient symbols, their esoteric meanings remain primarily unchanged throughout each script.

Runes Return to Their Original Use

When the runic alphabet moved to its final form of 27 characters in the Middle Ages, Latin was also introduced in Scandinavia. Yet it remained a foreign writing practice until the 16th century. This meant runic script remained popular for official memorials and records of important occurrences. Likewise, it was widely used for writing diaries and practicing magic or divination. This was especially true in Iceland, with its Rune Poems and manuscripts written in Medieval runes up to the 19th century. Moreover, Sweden mostly used runic calendars until that same period. Additionally, knowledge of their magical and divinatory uses has been preserved throughout history due to the 16th century's development of Runology.

Runology

The runes have been used and studied for divination purposes for a far longer time than the tarot has. Their use tracks back at least 2,000 years. The study of the runes began in the 16th century with the specialized branch of German linguistics known as runology. As mentioned in the previous chapter, the academic study of the runes started with the Swedish polymath JohannesBureus. Bureus considered the runes as tools for magic and divination handed down the generations from his Old Norse ancestors. He even went on to create his esoteric interpretation of the runes. While Bureus may have been the first runologist, he was not the last. This way, the runic script and the hidden meaning of the runes have carried on to the modern day.

Now that you understand the history and application of runes, it is time to infuse the magic, rituals, and wisdom of Runelore into your life. Subsequent chapters will teach you to use these timeless symbols' legendary might and wisdom to access your intuition.

3

Elder Futhark

As the oldest known runic alphabet, the Elder Futhark is a powerful source of knowledge and understanding. It forms the basis for all other runic scripts and contains 24 unique characters with distinct meanings. Ages-old runes were used by cultures worldwide to communicate with each other and access divine knowledge. This chapter explains their meanings and guides how to interpret them in your rune casts. Furthermore, these symbols may still help connect you to universal energies for spiritual growth and insight.

The Ætts of the Elder Futhark

The ancient Elder Futhark alphabet is divided into three distinct groups of eight runes, collectively known as ættir or "clans" in Old Norse. These clans have strong linkages to each other and can be used to form connections between past and present. Each group is rich in symbolic meaning, depicting ancient Norse gods, concepts, and beliefs. As such, the three ættir of the Elder Futhark includes the following:

- Freyr/Freyja's Ætt
- Heimdall's Ætt
- Týr's Ætt

Per ætt, which translates to 'family,' is a group of runes assigned to a specific god from the Norse pantheon. Fascinatingly, the name of each god matches the first letter of their corresponding set of runes—the Elder Futhark. Learn more about this magical language by exploring its different ættir and their divine rulers.

Freyr/Freyja's Ætt

The two powerful twins of Norse mythology, Freyr and Freyja, rule the first eight runes of the Elder Futhark. Freyr and Freyja, children of Njord, belong to the Vanir pantheon. This class of Norse gods is associated with wisdom, fertility, and the ability to see into the future.

Freyr means "Lord" in Old Norse and is the god of fertility. He was one of the most revered gods among both the Norse and Germanic people. As the god of fertility, Freyr had power over anything that grew, which is why he was so revered and prayed to by the Norse and Germanic peoples. Meanwhile, Freyja means "Lady" in Old Norse and is the goddess of love and beauty, sex and war, gold and fertility. She is also the goddess of seiðr *(seidr)*, the Old Norse word for a type of magic that could see into the future and influence it.

Freyr and Freyja's set of runes is known as the ætt of the nurturer - a representation of life, love, happiness, and joy. Like tarot cards, runes also have corresponding meanings. Yet, their connotations depend on whether upright or merkstave (reversed). Merkstave meaning is not the exact opposite of the original interpretation; think of it as a shadow to its light. Not all runes carry a merkstave, though, since some are impossible to tell if they are right side up or upside down. For rune casting, we will explore the eight runes of Freyr/Freyja's Ætt and discuss their light and dark meanings. Additionally, most Norse religions view divination as acquiring insight into one's personal growth rather than trying to predict future events. As such, knowledge about Norse mythology can help parse these runes better.

Fehu (ᚠ)

The rune fehu is connected to the Norse god Freyr and the goddess Freyja. Also, it serves as a reminder that success can be achieved through hard work and effort rather than solely relying on luck. It also symbolizes abundance, good fortune, and the potential for growth in various areas of life. Furthermore, numerous interpretations of fehu involve energy, foresight, creation, and destruction. In other words, it represents the power to transform a present situation into something greater. Ultimately, fehu stands for hope, wealth, and joy that can be attained when we take the necessary steps toward prosperity.

Fehu, when reversed in casting, indicates a loss due to one's actions or behavior. It can refer to losing material possessions, assets, or self-esteem interpreted as greed, discord among relationships, and burnout. In addition, fehu's negative form could symbolize poverty, cowardice, or being bound by obligations. All this serves as a reminder to take caution in life and our decisions, which could have greater implications than intended.

Ūruz (ᚢ)

The rune ūruz is the second in Freyr/Freyja's Ætt and dates back to the Proto-Germanic language. This form symbolizes physical strength and untamed potential. When appearing face-up in a divinatory casting, it signifies tremendous energy and hidden power. Conversely, its merkstave form carries implications of weakness, misdirection, obsession, lust, and violence. Depending on where it appears with other runes, ūruz may signify understanding, wisdom, sexuality, sexual desire, or maleness. When interpreted through these various lenses, ūruz suggests positivity. Yet, unexpected changes are coming into your life due to self-formation and a need for mindful actions.

Thurisaz (Þ)

The 'th' of the Futhark, Thurisaz, is believed to mean 'giant,' as in the mythical creature. Norse gods were often embroiled in a war with these powerful beings. Ragnarök was sparked by fire giants siding with Loki and Surtr against Odin and the Æsir at the apocalyptic battle. Interestingly, not all deities shared this hostility; Thor was half-giant and Odin's eldest son. Furthermore, giants have often been associated with wisdom, strength, and hidden knowledge, symbols of divine power that could explain why gods so fiercely regarded them.

Moreover, the rune Thurisaz is steeped in history and speaks to the power of duality. It is strongly associated with magical symbolism, representing the forces of connection and opposition within the universe. These opposing forces can be used for constructive purposes. However, they can lead to conflict, defensiveness, or destruction if unchecked. As a representation of vitality and sexual energy, Thurisaz is believed to symbolize fertility and uncontrolled aspirations. Understanding this intricate relationship between positive and negative points can unlock more powerful aspects of their own will.

On merkstave meaning, its presence in a reading can be seen as a warning of the potential for betrayal, malice, hatred, or lies to enter one's life. As such, it is associated with feelings of vulnerability. Likewise, it could be interpreted as a sign that something is amiss in one's environment or with a relationship.

Those looking for further insight might use it to evaluate if there are any negative influences present in their lives that need to be addressed. Additionally, the rune has been used for centuries by those seeking guidance about their future and possible outcomes. Thus, providing yet another layer of significance when it appears in readings.

Ansuz (ᚨ)

Represented by the letter 'a', Ansuz is the rune signifying insight and connection to one's spiritual self. It can be interpreted as a blessing bestowed upon you or an indication to accept divine advice. Commonly thought to refer to Odin himself, this symbol of knowledge and wisdom carries omens of good health, truth, and harmony. Additionally, this ancient symbol is known for its spiritual guidance, symbolizing that one should heed the advice bestowed upon them by the gods. Ansuz has also been connected to creative communication, indicating that it may benefit those looking to create or engage with their audience meaningfully. Yet, when its interpretation is reversed, it may warn of misunderstanding, manipulation, and negative feelings such as vanity and arrogance.

Raidho (ᚱ)

The 'r' of the Futhark, Raidho, symbolizes a journey of physical travel and transformation. It indicates that you are about to embark on a journey leading to personal growth and evolution. This rune encourages decisive action toward making the best next move. Also, it relates to the rhythms of life and how your rhythm can fit within them. Furthermore, tracing this rune in grounding rituals is believed to help clear away any negative energy preventing you from furthering your journey. Ultimately, raidho speaks to the beauty of discovery and changing perspectives that comes with traveling life's path.

For its merkstave interpretation, raidho suggests a time of disruption and impending crisis. This could be interpreted as a warning that something is about to disturb or halt your progress or journey in life or even foreshadow death itself. In Norse mythology, raidho was associated with journeys, communication, and traveling great distances. It was also seen as being related to death and the afterlife. This connection to fate and destiny makes this rune important in divination and understanding life events.

Kaunan (<)

Kaunan, the 'k' rune of the Elder Futhark, is closely associated with healing. This interpretation of the rune emerged during a period of magical and spiritual practices in Scandinavia. The rune was believed to give strength and courage to those who sought its aid in recovering from sickness or injury. By looking more deeply into its meaning, kaunan can be interpreted as an invitation to boldly move toward physical and mental health. Much like the Kenaz (torch), which many prefer, this original k-rune signifies new possibilities and a rediscovery of inner strength.

The appearance of Kaunan in reading or interaction can bring about profound shifts in energy and decisions. As such, it can signify both positive and negative outcomes. Likewise, it is associated with revelation, knowledge, creativity, clearing vision, and new energy sources, allowing you to create the life you want. On the shadow side, however, Kaunan signifies false hope, instability, loss of illusion, lack of creativity, and coming disease or illness. It could also portend a breakup or feeling exposed. Considering this symbol's aspects can help interpret your readings and uncover potential personal changes ahead.

Gebo (X)

First rune on the runic alphabet symbol after 'futhark,' Gebo, is derived from the 'g' phoneme and is translated to 'gift.' This rune signifies an equilibrium between giving and receiving. Yet, it is not limited to material things. Instead, it includes emotional and spiritual gifts exchanged in relationships and business contracts. Moreover, it stands for a transfer of energy which can be beneficial or detrimental depending on how it is used. Thus, gebo symbolizes the significance of balancing generosity with assertiveness.

In the context of divination, Gebo can denote an offer or gift-giving, with an expectation of something in return. It may also suggest that an individual has given too much, leading to feelings of loneliness, greed, or obligation. However, when lying in opposition to other runes, Gebo changes its meaning to indicate a loss of equilibrium. As such, it can be either self-sacrificing oneself excessively or having to make payments through no fault of your own. In these cases, it can be viewed as a sign of bribery.

Wunjo (ᚹ)

Wunjo is the 24th rune in the Elder Futhark. It has been used to represent both the letters 'w' and 'v,' with its meaning connected to joy, love, fertility, spiritual reward, and community. Likewise, it brings comfort, pleasure, success, harmony, and prosperity. But it is also important to remember that too much of a good thing can be bad. Hence, avoid becoming overly excessive when interpreting wunjo.

Aside from that, Wunjo is believed to originate in Viking culture, which associated it with the god Odin and his infamous rage. Subsequently, its merkstave version of this rune is a sign of despair. Likewise, it is related to misguided decisions or alienation from others. In extreme cases, it can represent uncontrolled anger, an out-of-control frenzy, and even intoxication or possession. This rune is said to indicate a state of confusion and mindlessness. It can also signify a lack of control over one's actions and a disconnection from reality.

With Wunjo, we come to the end of the ætt of the first degree, ruled over by the "Lord" Frey and the "Lady" Freyja. Like the two gods who rule over it, this ætt is composed of opposites. In fact, three pairs represent each rune in the word Futhark. Fehu and Ūruz, the domesticated and the wild. Then, Thurisaz and Ansuz, the giants and the gods. Meanwhile, Raidho and Kaunan, the journey (experience) and the sickness (knowledge). Moving on to the next aett of the Elder Futhark, let us explore more aspects this ancient alphabet has to offer.

Heimdall's Ætt

Heimdall is described in Norse mythology as the watchman of Asgard, the realm of the gods and its guardian. Odin gave Heimdall the task, the chief god he served faithfully, to sound a horn known as Gjallarhorn when Ragnarök begins. This serves as an alert that Ragnarök is starting and a warning to all beings in Asgard. Along with his role as watchman of Asgard, Heimdall also guards Bifröst, an enchanted rainbow bridge connecting Midgard (the realm of mortal men) and Asgard. To counterbalance, Heimdall's role in guarding heaven's entrance is Móðguðr (Mordgud). As such, Móðguðr is a maiden etin who stands guard over Gjallarbrú. This is a bridge crossing the river Gjöll which leads to hell in Norse mythology. Ergo, Móðguðr tasked with guiding those who have recently died across it so they cannot return to the land of the living.

The guardian of heaven and the guardian of hell ruling over this ætt symbolizes change, growth, and transformation. These runes can help clarify your purpose and strength to overcome life's challenges. Through these eight runes, you can decipher deeper meanings in your surroundings and use them to guide and inform your decisions. Learning to read and interpret these symbols allows you to uncover hidden layers of understanding that provide insight into our lives. Thus, this set of runes is much more than a simple divinatory tool; it is a gateway to self-discovery and enlightenment.

Hagalaz (H)

The first rune in this set is Hagalaz (h), which means 'hail.' This rune symbolizes nature's destructive, creative force and things outside our control. The way to think of the three ættir is as three 'levels' of a life's journey. The first ætt deals with the external and internal influences that create the individual. This second set, sometimes called Hell's Ætt, is about testing and challenging to help further the individual grow and develop. This is captured from the first rune—Hagalaz—which symbolizes tempering, testing, or enduring a trial leading to heightened inner harmony if the storm can be weathered first.

Hagalaz is the second rune that does not have a merkstave form. As with Gebo, this does not mean that Hagalaz cannot be interpreted in a 'dark' way, but that it is another rune that lies in opposition (if it falls with the rune skew or sideways in a casting). If it lies in opposition, Hagalaz warns of an impending natural disaster or catastrophe of some kind or form. It can also mean losing power or feeling powerless to control the pain and suffering in your life.

Naudiz (ᛏ)

The 'n' of the Elder Futhark, Naudiz, signifies a time of need and distress. It is an obstacle to success, prompting you to tap into your inner strength and show greater resolve. Naudiz challenges you to control your emotions and act with poise during strife.

These traits define endurance and determination in life. This powerful symbol implies survival and provides a unique opportunity to hone patience in challenging moments. With its origins firmly planted in Norse mythology, naudiz stands out as a representation of the journey towards triumph.

On the other hand, Naudiz suggests confinement and a lack of autonomy. It can come in various forms, from arduous labor to deprivation and deprivation of essential things. This could also be interpreted as unfulfilled needs, financial instability, and almost unbearable hunger. In extreme cases, Naudiz merkstave can even signify death from starvation or poverty. To further explain this concept, in Icelandic culture, it was believed that when someone had surpassed their limits or faced mortifying conditions, their spirit would turn into a wraith known as a 'naudhiz.' As such, they will be forced to live out the remainder of their existence in hideous poverty and deprivation.

Isaz (I)

With the meaning of "ice," Isaz (i) is the rune of challenge, frustration, and seeking a way to overcome them. The imagery of freezing is the best way to interpret this rune. As such, Isaz indicates that you are physically or psychologically in a state of frozen action, a block. To rectify this, take some time out to seek clarity from within and prepare for what is to come as you get *'unstuck.'* Isaz is a rune that reinforces the meaning or interpretation of the other runes connected to it in the cast. Also, Isaz has no merkstave form. Yet, if lying in opposition, it can be interpreted as selfish behavior or an over-indulgence in sensual pleasures. Likewise, it can be a forewarning of a possible betrayal of trust or treachery or that plots are afoot against you.

Jēran (ᛃ)

The J-rune, or *"Jēran,"* symbolizes reaping the rewards of your efforts. Likewise, it can be interpreted to mean peace, prosperity, happiness, hope, and success. Sometimes, it is referred to as "jera" and represents the continuous cycle of life in the universe. As a positive omen, it is believed that when this rune appears, it honors good fortune and could bring abundance in all areas of life. Additionally, Jēran carries with it the meaning of a *"good harvest"* or *"good year."* Hence, it signifies greater assurance for those around them that their future will be filled with plenty.

Aside from that, Jēran has no merkstave version. Yet, this rune is often seen as a sign of misfortune and can portend delays or plan disruptions. Those with this rune in opposition can expect their good fortune to be unceremoniously reversed without warning. It also shows that timing is everything when making meaningful changes. Also, it emphasizes the importance of being prepared for the unexpected.

Eihwaz (ᛇ)

Representing *'y'*, Eihwaz stands for *'yew tree'* and is the start of the second half of the Elder Futhark. Symbolically, it represents Yggdrasil, the world tree. As such, it symbolizes strength, dependability, trustworthiness, and reliability. In Norse mythology, this rune is associated with enlightenment and protection. Eihwaz is a sign that you are on the right path to achieving your goals and can attain them with effort. Then, in its inverted form (merkstave), Eihwaz can indicate confusion or weakness. Subsequently, it signifies a need to seek clarity and gain inner strength. Ultimately, this rune serves as a reminder of humankind's potential for self-discovery and growth.

Perthro (⌡)

Although the precise meaning of Perthro, represented by the *'p'* of the Elder Futhark, is unknown, its significance is known to be a lot cup. Warriors used this ancient dice box to cast lots to determine their fate before a battle. Perthro is associated with Orlog, an old Norse term for *"fate"* or the fundamental principles of the universe. It represents secrecy, hidden knowledge, and understanding of our destiny. Some interpret it as determining one's path, while others consider it a sign of uncertainty. In addition, it is said that casting lots with this rune served as a way for Northern Europeans to communicate with their gods during times of crisis and upheaval. Yet, in merkstave readings, perthro suggests the feeling of addiction and loneliness. For instance, it can be seen as a sign of a lack of progress, deep unhappiness, or emotional malaise.

Algiz (Y)

In the ancient runic alphabet, Algiz or *'z,'* symbolizes protection and stands for the spiritual bond between mortals and deities. It serves as a shield to ward off evil forces and assists in connecting to one's higher self. Likewise, it may point out an awakening or divine favor in one's life. Furthermore, it denotes the importance of controlling energy to avoid potential pitfalls. Conversely, when its inverted form appears in a cast, it indicates hidden dangers or losing access to the spiritual realm. Thus, it is a sign of rejection, suggesting something should be changed soon.

Sowilō (ϟ)

Heimdall's Ætt's final rune, sowilō, means *'sun'* and signifies success, accomplishment, and honor. It also speaks to wholeness, positive transformation, and the power to realize ambitions. Connecting your higher self to your innermost thoughts and feelings, this rune stands as a reminder that the sun's energy can be used to clear away negative influences. As such, it is an emblem of spiritual cleansing and renewal. Furthermore, sowilō is believed to grant access to greater awareness and intuition, allowing for a deeper understanding of one's existence.

Sowilō, in merkstave, suggests a lack of connection with our spiritual selves. It could signify delusions, misguidedness, and actions resulting from bad counsel or advice. When interpreted as an omen, it could mean that one will face failure in achieving their goals if they are not well thought out. Further, this rune also signifies a disconnection from nature. As such, it is a blockage to our inherent natural wisdom and connection to the energetic powers within us.

As we have seen, the second set of the Elder Futhark, known as Heimdall's Ætt, delves into the *"Great Trials of Life."* These runes bear the weighty truth of self-development and our connection to destiny. They speak of a journey that culminates in sowilō, an inner strength that grants us the ability to choose our path. With this knowledge, we can become fully formed, successful individuals, conquering life's great trials.

Týr's Ætt

Týr, the god of war and sacrifice, justice and order, and patron of warriors, governs the final set of runes in the Elder Futhark. He was revered for his cosmic judgment and moral values and encouraged spiritual achievement. Connected to this is the belief that he had a hand in the mythical heroes from legends or myths. In fact, he is remembered as a symbol of established order and atonement. As such, it makes sense why these eight runes have been placed under his protection, for they represent some form of struggle, resolution, or peacekeeping within society. Thus concludes our journey into defining the great symbols that make up the Elder Futhark.

Tiwaz (ᛏ)

Tiwaz, also known as the rune of Tyr, is a symbol of justice and honor. It stands for a victory achieved through taking the right course of action. Also, it encourages its followers to take time for self-reflection. Likewise, to analyze and identify their strengths and weaknesses. The courage this rune highlights means making difficult decisions with the potential for personal sacrifice to win and reach success. With perseverance and dedication, its followers will eventually emerge victorious.

For the merkstave of Tiwaz, it signifies difficulty in progress and stagnation. Often, it is characterized by an imbalance between thought and action. It is also a warning sign of blocked creativity, paralyzing self-sacrificing, or over-analysis. Additionally, it can be interpreted as the diminishing of passion due to a lack of communication or injustice that leads to separation. Understanding this rune can greatly help personal growth. For instance, it reveals blind spots and shows how one's life may need adjustment to restore harmony and balance.

Berkanen (ᛒ)

The second rune in Týr's Ætt is berkanen. Representing the letter 'b,' this rune means 'birch' and signifies fertility, birth, and growth. It is a rune of liberation or regeneration, renewal, and the start of something new. Plus, it could also mean that new love is about to come into your life, romantic or otherwise, and that prosperous times are ahead. Berkanen merkstave is a sign of problems, especially those related to family or domestic issues. Likewise, it is a sign of anxiety or carelessness, abandonment, or losing control. Finally, berkanen merkstave warns of stagnation, being sterile (infertile), or deception.

Ehwaz (ᛖ)

Carrying the meaning of *'horse,'* Ewhaz is the *'e'* of the Elder Futhark. Symbolizing movement, progress, and development achieved, it inspires collaboration and trusts in relationships. It also represents a strong connection to those around it. Whether for marriage or partnership, loyalty and faithfulness are associated with this rune. Additionally, ehwaz is a sign of good fortune and freedom, as it could symbolize success after a journey or a change in direction. This rune, therefore, serves as an affirmation that all changes are positive ones.

On the merkstave side, ehwaz signifies restlessness or unease that must be addressed. This rune symbolizes the need for balance and careful consideration when changing one's life. The so-called merkstave is seen as a cautionary note. As such, it can portend unhappiness caused by hastily made choices or betrayals of trust. The key with this rune is to ensure that any changes are done slowly, thoughtfully, and in a way that honors both the past and future.

Mannaz (ᛗ)

One of the few runes where you can immediately recognize the English word derived from it is mannaz. The *'m'* phoneme means *'man'* or *'humankind.'* It symbolizes the self, your perception and treatment of others, and their views of you. Mannaz is a sign of friendship and hostility, depicting order in society and structure in the divine. As well as being associated with intelligence and creativity, this rune indicates that aid or assistance will soon enter your life. Additionally, mannaz has traditionally been used as a talisman to bring luck to its wearer. Its connection with humanity affords it extra spiritual power when used to invoke good fortune and protection.

As for the merkstave interpretation of mannaz, it implies mortality and human frailties like depression, delusion, and blindness. This symbol speaks to the darker nature of our thoughts. As such, these thoughts include manipulation, deceit, or cunning with malicious purpose. If this rune appears in your casting, it could represent a warning not to expect any help or guidance in what you seek to know.

Laguz (ᛚ)

The letter '*l,*' laguz, means '*lake*' or '*water*' and signifies healing, fertility, and renewal. It captures the flow of water, such as with the tides of the sea, and symbolizes the energy of life and growth in an organic way. Laguz represents the power of imagination, dreams, and fantastic mysteries. Likewise, it shows the hidden depths of this world and the one below it (the underworld). Finally, it can be seen as a sign of success or of acquiring something you have been seeking, but with the equivalent exchange of a price paid.

In terms of its merkstave form, laguz indicates impending changes, often of uncertain nature. It can manifest as an unwise decision, stagnancy in life, or even a mental disorder. Though not consistently negative, it may indicate an approaching period of difficulty. Yet, it may represent an opportunity to confront fears and take risks that could lead to personal growth and transformation.

Inguz (ᛜ)

Inguz, the '*ŋ*' phoneme, is the rune representing the god Ing. This is an older name for Freyr, the god of Earth. Inguz is a sign of fertility for men, of growing internally, or of a time for rest and recovery. It represents shared virtues or common sense, family bonds, and the warmth of humankind. If inguz appears in your casting, this is a sign that you should listen to your inner self and are ready to close off loose ends and head in a new life direction. However, unlike other runes, inguz has no merkstave form when lying in opposition. Instead, if interpreted, it suggests the idea of effort without any apparent change or tangible reward.

Dagaz (ᛞ)

With dagaz or *'d'*, it carries the meaning of *'day'* and symbolizes a time of awakening, heightened awareness, or an upcoming breakthrough. It is a sign of clarity that breaks through the uncertainty of the night that came before. Dagaz indicates that it is time for you to get planning for your next adventure or get ready to embark on one. Plus, it is a sign that you have the willpower to enforce the change or transformation you want to see in your life. Likewise, dagaz is the rune of hope and happiness, living your ideal life and being secure and confident of your path forward. If this rune appears in your casting, interpret it as meaning that a time of growing and releasing or balancing opposite forces is upon you.

Like ingaz before it, dagaz also signals the end of a chapter by reaching your limits or being blind to something that influences you. Sometimes, dagaz also points to being in an entirely helpless position. Connected to this idea is the Norse concept of wyrd. As such, it is a belief that fates beyond their control predetermine one's destiny. Whatever actions are taken will shape the outcome, but ultimately, one's ultimate path is out of their hands.

Othala (ᛟ)

Othala is the 24th rune of the Elder Futhark rune system. This rune holds great significance for those who practice Nordic spirituality. The symbol of othala is associated with prosperity, wealth, and inheritance. It represents a connection to one's past and family legacy. For this reason, othala often acts as a reminder to stay grounded in traditional values while embarking on new experiences. Besides that, it is seen as a protector during the transition, providing stability and security in times of change.

The card of othala, when reversed, is associated with being out of touch with one's culture and customs. This may lead to feeling disconnected or a sense of loss. It may also signify difficulties finding success due to bad luck or unfair discrimination. Lastly, othala could point to poverty, displacement, slavery, or feeling held captive by something.

4

Younger Futhark

The Younger Futhark, also known as *"Viking Runes" or* the *"Scandinavian Runes,"* was the successor to the Elder Futhark alphabet. This transition was seen in Scandinavia during the 7th to 8th centuries AD, with the Elder Futhark slowly being replaced by its successor in the 9th century. During this same period, Proto-Norse gave way to Old Norse. As such, it provided an opportunity for further linguistic and literary development. Subsequently, it has strongly influenced Scandinavian culture. As well as serving as an essential writing system, runes were used for magic purposes and are still respected and valued today.

Moreover, the Younger Futhark was a more condensed form of the Elder Futhark. As such, it consists of only 16 runes as opposed to its predecessor's 24. This reduction in characters was concurrent with an increase in the number of phonemes used by the Scandinavian people. Used throughout the Viking Age (793-1066 AD), it experienced a steady decline. That is due to Scandinavia integrating Christian ideologies alongside the Latin script. Despite this waning usage, Young Futhark runes were still employed in an auxiliary capacity. Usually, they are utilized for magical and divinatory practices or secret messages inscribed as memorials. With its decline came a shift away from runes as the central writing system of Germanic and Scandinavian peoples, heralding a new era within these societies.

Tracing its roots back to the Elder Futhark, the Younger Futhark runes were used in divination and rune casting. Likewise, it served as a written language for ancient northern European societies. There are two main branches of the Younger Futhark. These two include the Danish long-branch and Swedish or Norwegian short-twig runes, further divided into Hälsinge Runes. This chapter outlines the Younger Futhark's origins, history, and evolution from its earliest beginnings. Plus, it will provide invaluable insight into how this powerful symbolic system can be used to divine our future.

History of the Younger Futhark

Late in 700 AD, the Viking Age began. During this time, there was a mass change in the world. For instance, Scandinavian and Germanic people, or the Vikings, conquered much of Europe and Great Britain. With this age of expansion and exploration also came a change in the language of these raiders, pillagers, and conquerors from Proto-Norse to Old Norse. Also, ancient northern cultures shifted from the obscure Elder Futhark, used for personal runemasters, to the Younger Futhark, a much more widespread and accessible writing system.

As literacy flourished among the Norse people in the 9th century AD, so did the use of the Younger Futhark. Though there was some overlap between the Elder and Younger Futhark symbols from 650 to 800 AD, the Elder Futhark eventually succumbed to its successor. The Younger Futhark was better suited for the times. Also, the Vikings utilized it in matters both serious and light. As such, it was used in trade documents, diplomatic correspondences, poems, jests, and personal messages.

Long-Branch Runes

While the Younger Futhark is the name for the runic script, a few variations have been found. The oldest of these is known as the Danish long-branch runes. This branch-rune originated in and around modern-day Denmark, the ancestral home of the Danes. Primarily, they were carved on stone and are the more complicated versions of the Younger Futhark runes. Yet, they are still simpler than those of the Elder Futhark because they only have one vertical line known as a *'stave.'*

Short-Twig Runes

Developing after the Danish long-branch runes came to the short-twig version of the Younger Futhark runic script. Primarily used in Sweden and Norway, these runes were easier to carve. Also, compared to their long-branch counterparts, they were formed without a full vertical stave. During the end of the Viking Age, short-twig runes became more popular, continuing in use even into medieval times. Besides that, they can be considered the short-hand or cursive version of the runes. Due to that, scribes and traders favored them, as they were easier and quicker to carve. Moreover, they are also known as the Rök runes. As such, they are named after the Rök runestone, the longest runic inscription engraved on the stone.

The Runes of the Younger Futhark

Runes were used to cast spells and were believed to represent power, protection, and good luck. These runes were inscribed on amulets and jewelry the Viking people wore. Furthermore, Norse mythology often describes the runes as a language the gods gave to humanity. The Codex Sangallensis 878 is an illustrated manuscript estimated to date back to around 830 AD. As such, it contains 24 stanzas related to the runes of the Younger Futhark.

This codex, recorded in a monastery in Switzerland, contains many alphabets of the ancient world. On page 321 is the Abecedarium Nordmannicum, three lines presenting the runes of the Younger Futhark. On the same page are the runes of the Anglo-Saxon Futhorc. However, this recording does not give us an explanation of the meanings of the runes. For that, we looked to the Icelandic Rune Poem recorded in the 15th century and translated into English by B. Dickens in 1915.

Let us delve deeper into the runes and the messages they hold. The Icelandic Rune Poem offers excellent insight into the meaning of each rune in the Younger Futhark. Also, it provides an interpretation for us to ponder and orient our castings. Taking the time to contemplate their meanings can open new perspectives on life's questions.

Freyr/Freyja's Ætt

As we mentioned earlier, the ætt ruled over by Freyr and Freyja lost its final two members as the runic alphabet transformed from the Elder to the Younger Futhark. Two runes, ansuz and kaunan changed in shape. Meanwhile, the rest remained the same, although their pronunciation differed from their counterparts. This is because the spoken language of the Elder Futhark was Proto-Norse. In contrast, the language of the Younger Futhark, the Scandinavian Runes, was Old Norse, the language of the Vikings.

Fé (ᚠ)

"Source of discord among kinsmen
and fire of the sea
and path of the serpent."
(Icelandic Rune Poem Verse 1)

Younger Futhark's *'f'* and *'v,'* fé represents wealth and abundance. During the Viking Age, *'cattle'* and *'wealth'* were considered the same, so this sign was highly regarded. Fé remained intact with its original meaning throughout both Elder and Younger Futhark eras. Forging a link between physical and spiritual well-being, it also has strong ties to potential success or happiness if cast upright. However, if reversed, it can represent a failure or significant loss. Yet, it still offers wisdom on preventing disaster in this context. In addition to this significance, fé is often connected with spiritual growth and prosperity, signifying the reaping of the rewards for hard work and dedication.

Úr (ᚢ)

> "Lamentation *of the clouds*
> and ruin the hay-harvest
> and abomination of the shepherd."
> **(Icelandic Rune Poem Verse 2)**

The Younger Futhark rune ᚢ, also known as úr, holds a spectrum of meanings from *'shower'* to *'iron'* and even *'rain.'* Yet, it contrasts with its elder version, ūruz, which means 'wild ox.' There have been two widely accepted interpretations of ᚢ in the Elder Futhark. One is ūruz *(aurochs)*, and the other is ūrą *(water)*. Old English and the Anglo-Saxon futhorc stay true to its úr rune's meaning of *'auroch.'* But when considering Old Norse and the Younger Futhark, ᚢ takes on a new interpretation of úr *(denoting 'rain')*. If you want to explore this rune's significance in more detail, let us unpack its enigmatic úr form. Likewise, let us learn how it can influence your divination readings.

Upright Úr is often seen as a symbol of new beginnings and potential. When upright, it signs fertility and signals that blessings may come your way or something unexpected could arise. On the other hand, in its reversed form, úr conveys misguided force or energy and serves as a reminder to stay vigilant. Those bearing this rune are cautioned to take heed of their surroundings to protect themselves from sudden danger.

Þhurs (þ)

> *"Torture of women*
> *and cliff-dweller*
> *and husband of a giantess."*
> **(Icelandic Rune Poem Verse 3)**

Thurs *(Þhurs)* is the Younger Futhark equivalent of Thurisaz *(þ)*. It carries the meaning of *'giant,'* representing the main opposition to the gods in Norse mythology. The interpretation of þhurs is similar to the Thurisaz of the Elder Futhark. This is the rune of brute strength and signifies conflict and vitality. If reversed in its merkstave form, it is a warning sign of impending danger or malice.

Óss (ᚯ)

> *"Aged Gautr*
> *and prince of Ásgarðr*
> *and lord of Vallhalla."*
> **(Icelandic Rune Poem Verse 4)**

Óss (ᚯ) is the Younger Futhark equivalent of the a-rune from the Elder Futhark, ansuz (ᚨ). They may look and sound different, but both are believed to represent Odin, or *'God'* in Norse mythology. As such, the óss rune is associated with communication, the ability to convey insight, wisdom, and good advice. In contrast, its merkstave is linked to deceit and manipulation through miscommunication or misunderstanding.

Reið (ᚱ)

> *"Joy of the horsemen*
> *and speedy journey*
> *and toil of the steed."*
> **(Icelandic Rune Poem Verse 5)**

Reið, or ræið in Old Norse, is the Younger Futhark's version of raidō. It carries the same runic shape, sound, and meaning as its Elder Futhark version. This is the rune of the journey or the quest for enlightenment, and it means *'riding'* in both the physical and metaphorical sense of movement. On its good side lies personal evolution through experience, while on its bad is a dislocation from the world's rhythm.

Kaun (ᚴ)

> *"Disease fatal to children*
> *and painful spot*
> *and abode of mortification."*
> **(Icelandic Rune Poem Verse 6)**

Replacing kaunan, the *'k'* rune of the Elder Futhark, is kaun, the *'k,' 'g,'* and *'ŋ'* of the Younger Futhark. Carrying the exact meaning of 'ulcer' and representing sickness and disease or the curing or avoidance thereof, Kaun is the rune of wisdom achieved through suffering. Though it is known for hardship, the rune Kaun also represents positive transformation and clarity of vision. When reversed in a casting, however, its meanings become more ominous. As such, it can be a warning of illness, feeling exposed to vulnerability, or lack of learning from suffering.

Heimdall's Ætt

As discussed in the preceding chapter, Heimdall's Ætt concerns beginnings and endings, transformation, and chaos. This second set of runes infers an entranceway to heaven, the underworld, and even other realms. Like the first ætt, two runes had been removed in the Younger Futhark. As such, these two are eihwaz (yew tree) and perthro (lot cup). Then, one rune from this ætt, Algiz (z-rune), was relocated to Týr's Ætt, being changed into its new R-rune form. Thus, the remaining five runes further explain the spiritual journey associated with this ætt.

Hagall (*)

"Cold grain
and a shower of sleet
and sickness of serpents."
(Icelandic Rune Poem Verse 7)

Hagall, formerly known as hagalaz (H) of the Elder Futhark, is a rune that symbolizes sudden change. It emphasizes the importance of learning from hardships. Likewise, it highlights accepting the tests and challenges that accompany personal growth. There is no negative interpretation associated with this rune. However, it can sometimes be interpreted as an omen of a pending disaster. The long-branch version of Hagall is '*,' while its short-twig variant is '/.' Lastly, its meaning remains unchanged, as it translates to 'hail.'

Nauðr (†)

"Grief of the bondmaid
and state of oppression
and toilsome work."
(Icelandic Rune Poem Verse 8)

Keeping the same runic shape as naudiz and the meaning of *'need'* or *'constraint,'* nauðr is much the same as its Elder Futhark equivalent. This includes the way to interpret it in your castings. It is the rune of necessity and difficulty. In its upright form, nauðr represents inner strength amidst distress or confusion. On the contrary, its merkstave form signifies want, poverty, or unmet emotional needs. Finally, the long-branch form of nauðr is '𐌵,' while the short-twig version is '𐌷.'

Íss (I)

> *"Bark of rivers*
> *and roof of the wave*
> *and destruction of the doomed."*
> **(Icelandic Rune Poem Verse 9)**

The single-stave rune of isaz remained unchanged in its evolution into íss. However, it did pick up another phoneme to represent along the way, standing for both the sounds *'i'* and *'e'* in the runic script of the Younger Futhark. Meaning *'ice'* is the rune of self-control and signifies seeking a way to overcome challenges and frustrations. As a single stave, íss has no merkstave form. Yet, if it lies in opposition, it could be a sign of betrayal, self-centered behavior, or over-indulgence in the world's pleasures.

Ár (ᛅ)

> *"Boon to men*
> *and good summer*
> *and thriving crops."*
> **(Icelandic Rune Poem Verse 10)**

Jēran *(ᛃ),* the j-rune of the Elder Futhark, has a fascinating past. Once meaning *'good harvest,'* it evolved into ár *(ᛅ),* which stands for *'plenty.'* Even more remarkable is its shift in pronunciation from representing the 'j' sound to 'a,' 'æ,' and 'e.' This transition from Proto-Germanic to Old Norse was likely the cause of this dramatic change. Additionally, the rune served several purposes throughout ancient history. For instance, it can mark important milestones by symbolizing natural elements.

While the rune shape and associated sounds might have undergone an evolution, the meaning of the rune remained the same. Like jēran before it, ár is the rune of good results from skill, knowledge, hard work, and good timing. In other words, it is the rune of reaping what you sow. In its upright form, ár represents success, happiness, or prosperity. With no merkstave form, ár is a sign of a possible setback, bad timing, or a reversal of luck or fortune when in opposition. Also, the long-branch form of ár is '↑,' while the short-twig version is '↓.'

Sól (ᛋ)

> *"Shield of the clouds*
> *and shining ray*
> *and destroyer of ice."*
> **(Icelandic Rune Poem Verse 11)**

As the Elder Futhark had sowilō (ᛋ) to represent the 's' sound, so does the Younger Futhark have sól (ᛋ). Both mean 'sun,' but the younger version had an added meaning. In comparison, sowilō represents the elemental force of the sun's energy. Then, sól is the personification of the sun in the form of the goddess Sól. Regardless, it does not change how it is interpreted in your castings but adds to its meaning, as the sun goddess resides in this rune.

Moreover, sól is the rune of success, achievement, and wholeness. In its upright form, this rune indicates positive change and that you are on track to achieving your life goals. Yet, in opposition, as it has no merkstave form, sól indicates a disconnection from your purpose or a risk of losing sight of your goals. This rune's short-twig version is ' ⸌.'

With the rune of the sun comes the end of the second ætt. Now that Heimdall's five runes are covered, it is time to turn to the final set of the Younger Futhark.

Týr's Ætt

Losing the most runes out of the three, Týr's Ætt gained one back as the z-rune transformed and moved from Heimdall's Ætt to the end of the alphabet. From that, Týr's Ætt in the Younger Futhark consists of five runes. Ruled over by Týr, the one-handed god of cosmic judgment and moral values, this ætt deals with the forces of the cosmos. As the final part of the runic alphabet's magical journey, Týr's Ætt symbolizes the knowledge gained from the trials of the previous ætt. Aside from that, it also represents this knowledge being put to use beyond the self to better the family, the community, or even human society at large. Through this, one may become in tune with the cosmic laws of love, collaboration, responsibility, and contribution to the future of our planet. While on this journey, the individual becomes enlightened and reaches spiritual fulfillment.

Týr (↑)

"God, with one hand
and leavings of the wolf
and prince of temples."
(Icelandic Rune Poem Verse 12)

Týr (ᛏ) serves as a reminder of the Norse god, Týr, the patron god of justice and heroic glory. It denotes victory, honors, and a need to define strengths and refine intentions. Its merkstave meaning warns against over-analyzing, sacrificing too much of oneself, or being out of touch with one's purpose. A long-branch version, 'ᛏ,' and a short-twig variant, 'ᛐ,' exist for this rune. Additionally, Týr is similar in shape and meaning to its equivalent in the Elder Futhark, tiwaz (ᛏ). This ancient symbol is a powerful reminder to stay true to one's course, no matter the outcome.

Björk (ᛒ)

"Leafy twig
and little tree
and fresh young shrub."
(Icelandic Rune Poem Verse 13)

The second rune of Týr's Ætt is björk (ᛒ). Likewise, it is called bjarkan or bjarken and is the evolution of the Elder Futhark's berkanen (ᛒ). Having the same rune shape, it also carries the same meaning as its descendant in the Younger Futhark. Björk represents the voiced 'b' and unvoiced 'p' while berkanen only stands for 'b.' This rune means 'birch,' a tree that symbolizes spring and rebirth. As such, björk is the rune of conception, gestation, and birth. Plus, it is the rune of feminine energy and divinity. When upright, it is a sign of renewal or the start of something new. However, lying in opposition is a sign of problems ahead or stagnation. Aside from that, björk does not have a short-twig version.

Maðr (ᛘ)

"Delight of man
and augmentation of the earth
and adorner of ships."
(Icelandic Rune Poem Verse 14)

With the removal of ehwaz, the e-rune of the Elder Futhark, maðr (ᛘ) is next in Týr's Ætt. Evolving from the Elder Futhark's mannaz (ᛗ), the meaning and the sound represented remained the same. Then, only the word and the runic shape change. With the meaning of *'man'* or *'human,'* maðr is the rune of human life and intelligence. It not only refers to humankind as a whole but also to the first man from Norse and Germanic creation myths, mannus. Our main source for mannus comes from Tacitus, one of Rome's historians who included the myth of mannus. This mannus is a Latinization of *'mannaz'* in his book Germania 10, published in 98 AD.

According to Tacitus, Mannus was the son of Tuisto, the divine ancestor of the Germanic peoples, who was the son of Earth. The children of Mannus are recorded in ancient songs of the Germanic people as the original ancestors of many early Germanic tribes. It is in the light of the original families of humanity with which you should view this rune as a symbol of the human family.

The runic symbol for maðr, ᛘ, is derived from algiz, ᛉ, the z- rune of the Elder Futhark. Algiz connotes *'protection,'* signifying a spiritual bond between humans and the gods. An upright appearance of maðr in your castings points to awareness, capability, support, or help. On the other hand, an inverted rendering of this symbol alludes to mortality or the difficulties faced by humankind. Moreover, maðr does not have a short-twig variant.

Lögr (ᛚ)

"Eddying stream
and broad Geysir
and the land of the fish."
(Icelandic Rune Poem Verse 15)

The evolution of laguz (ᛚ) from the Elder Futhark finds a similar form in lögr (ᛚ) of the Younger runic alphabet. Both runes carry the meaning of *'lake,' 'sea,'* or *'water,'* with the same runic shape and representing the same phoneme *(l)*. Lögr is the rune of life energy and purification. It symbolizes the washing away of unwanted or no longer-needed parts of ourselves as we *'cleanse'* the energy of our lives.

When cast in an upright form, it symbolizes that you are on the right path to reaching your goals. Akin to nature's equilibrium, this calls for a cost, a price to pay for the success you wish to gain. Conversely, if cast in a reversed or 'merkstave' form, it implies difficulties and uncertainty lie ahead. No short-twig version of lögr was indicated.

Yr (ᛦ)

"Bent bow
and brittle iron
and giant of the arrow."
(Icelandic Rune Poem Verse 16)

With the meaning of *'yew'* or, more specifically, *'bow made from a yew tree,'* yr (ᛦ) carries the same meaning as eihwaz (ᛇ) of the Elder. They are, however, different in their runic shape and the sounds they represent. Also, it is the recreation of the Elder Futhark's z-rune, algiz (ᛉ). Yr captures the change in how *'z'* was pronounced as Proto-Germanic evolved into Old Norse. The z phoneme became more of an *'r'* sound known as a voiced uvular trill, a hard, guttural *'r'* sound rolled with the back of the tongue. As such, it is written as *'R.'* Finally, yr (ᛦ) is an inversion of maðr (ᛘ), the life rune, often called the *'death rune.'* Besides that, this rune marks the only change of letter order the Futhark experienced as it evolved out of its elder form.

The Elder Futhark ends with the rune othala (ᛟ), the symbol of heritage or inheritance. It is a reminder to honor our ancestors by returning what was given to us and, in turn, passing it on. On the other hand, the Younger Futhark concludes its runes with Yr (ᛉ), a symbol representing death and rebirth. ᛉ is etched onto gravestones because this rune is thought to aid souls in their journey beyond the physical world. In addition, yr also signifies embarking on life's goals and gaining inner strength. Unlike the other runes, there is no 'merkstave' meaning associated with yr, nor does it boast any short-twig variant.

With the ancient rune of yr, representing death and resurrection, we complete Týr's Ætt and the Younger Futhark. This chapter detailed our knowledge of the Elder and Younger Futharks and how to interpret each rune in your readings. Now it is up to you to decide which version you prefer. The upcoming chapter will explore the fascinating Anglo-Saxon Futhorc and one of its main works, the *'Anglo-Saxon Rune Poem.'*

5

Anglo-Saxon Futhorc

The Elder Futhark was the original runic alphabet, representing Germanic languages in Northern Europe. Its evolution into the Younger Futhark around 200 AD marked the beginning of its use on the Scandinavian and European mainland, where Old Norse reigned supreme. A sister system to the Younger Futhark emerged to fit a foreign language in the British Isles. This system, known as the futhorc, comprises 33 runes used for Old English.

From the 5th to 12th centuries, Anglo-Saxon runes were ubiquitous and served as the main writing system for Old English. However, with Latin's dominance in the 7th century AD, runes gave way to their alphabetical counterpart. Nevertheless, futhorc remained popular for divination and protective spells until the 12th century.

The futhorc was more developed than its sister system, taking after its parent script by extending from 24 to 33 runes. In this chapter, readers will journey through this final main runic system. Plus, we will understand how it differs from its predecessor and sister alphabets.

History of the Anglo-Saxon Futhorc

In the mid-5th century, the Anglo-Saxon Migration marked a turning point in British history. The end of Roman rule over the British Isles in 410 AD and the emergence of the Anglo-Saxon culture and people were significant events in this period. As Rome's grip on Britain faltered, England was among the first regions to suffer its weakening influence. Without Roman protection, local tribes such as Britons and Celts rose against Roman provinces held in England. This led to a decline in Roman military presence on British soil until their departure.

On the arrival of the Angles, Saxons, and Jutes, they changed Britain's leadership landscape. As such, they swiftly claimed power by establishing kingdoms of their own. Before this power shift, British Celtic and Latin were widely spoken, with Latin alphabets used for writing. By the time several centuries had passed, Old English was established as England's primary language, accompanied by its distinct writing system known as Anglo-Saxon Futhorc. These developments positioned England at a significant crossroads of history, culture, and language.

Originating from West Germanic tribes, the Old English language had a variety of influences influencing its development. The Angles, Saxons, Jutes, and Frisians all contributed to what later became Old English. A version of the runic alphabet known as 'Anglo-Frisian' runes was also heavily influenced by the languages spoken in the areas mentioned.

The Latin alphabet eventually supplanted Old English and runic script towards the end of the 7th century. As Christianity spread throughout England, Latin soon replaced both as the language of written communication during this period. Even so, runes continued to be used for divination until the 11th century.

Various texts note how these modified runic alphabets were interpreted differently across cultures. For example, Anglo-Saxon runes were used differently than their Nordic variants. Some sources indicate they were even employed in anti-witchcraft spells and magical incantations. This further highlights how diverse yet nuanced rune symbols can become when adapted across varying contexts and geographical locations.

The Runes of the Futhorc

Like the other two runic scripts, futhorc split into three sets of runes known as ættir. Each set consists of eight runes governed by a god or goddess. In addition to being used for traditional divination purposes, these runes can also be used in protective spells and other magical practices. Furthermore, nine new runes were added to the back of the futhorc. As such, these provide insights into magical powers and their meanings, which can be explored further. Consequently, this section offers the opportunity to delve deeper into all three ættir and examine what the new runes offer.

Freyr/Freyja's Ætt

From ancient times, runes have been used to convey wisdom and teach lessons. The first set of runes in the journey of the runic alphabet, Freyr and Freyja's Ætt, is composed of opposing forces we encounter while growing up. It symbolizes the challenges a student has to endure when they begin their esoteric studies into runology. This cluster of runes reflects conflicts between domestication and freedom, gods versus demons, and light and darkness. Moreover, the " *Gift Rune*" and " *Glory Rune*" at the end of this ætt are not juxtapositions but rewards for hard work given to an initiate. A gift for the trials faced, and ultimately glory for the prize won (wisdom).

When it comes to understanding how futhorc differs from Elder Futhark or Younger Futhark, there is an Anglo-Saxon rune poem that provides explanations of each rune's meaning as our basis. This poem was written by Christian monk Ælfric, also known as "*Ælfric the Grammarian,*" in his manuscript *Cotton Otho B.x fol. 165a – 165b* around 8th or 9th century.

The knowledge within these runes can be used to educate us on how different symbols represent different stages of growth in life; it is an invaluable resource that can guide us through our initiation into life. With the runes showing our way, we can use them as tools to master life's challenges on our journey for wisdom and glory.

Feoh (ᚠ)

> *"Wealth is a comfort to all men;*
> *yet must every man bestow it freely,*
> *if he wishes to gain honor in the sight of the Lord."*
> **(Old English Rune Poem Verse 1)**

From the earliest days of our journey with the futhorc, there is a definite difference in the mood that comes through its poem compared to those crafted for the Younger Futhark. While Icelandic and Norwegian rune poems depict fé (ᚠ) as a "*cause of strife among men,*" its Old English counterpart interprets it as an equal comfort to all so long as they share it. This concept of mutual exchange presents a notable contrast with the idea of sacrifice conveyed by the previous runic poem.

Feoh (ᚠ) signifies its sister rune in the Younger Futhark and its ancestor in Elder Futhark while maintaining a similar form. It is also associated with *f* and *v* sounds, which can be heard from its earliest incarnation as fehu (ᚠ). Representing wealth, this rune symbolizes family support during our developmental years, reminding us that we eventually have to go forth and strive for our prosperity. To clarify this point, feoh represents our ambitions despite hardships and adversities.

Ur (ᚢ)

"The aurochs is proud and has great horns;
it is a very savage beast and fights with its horns;
a great ranger of the moors, it is a creature of mettle."
(Old English Rune Poem Verse 2)

The rune úr (ᚢ) of the Younger Futhark has roots in Norse mythology, signifying the power of self-formation and transformation. It speaks to the ability to use one's inner strength and change the course of life, providing an energizing potential when cast upright. Meanwhile, a merkstave reading denotes domination by external forces blocking growth. Connected to *'aurochs,'* an extinct wild ox species known for its strength and unpredictable nature, this rune provides a potent reminder that with self-determination comes great power.

Þorn (Þ)

"The thorn is exceedingly sharp,
an evil thing for any knight to touch,
uncommonly severe on all who sit among them."
(Old English Rune Poem Verse 3)

A place where the futhorc differs from both versions of the futhark is in the meaning of the Þ rune of the alphabet. Although it keeps the same sound and shape, Þ means *'thorn'* in Old English, whereas it means *'giant'* in Old Norse and Proto-Germanic. The runes thurisaz (Elder Futhark) and þhurs (Younger Futhark) were the runes of brute strength, as well as the connection and opposition between the giants (demons) and the gods. Þorn, however, is a rune of destruction and defense. It represents the sharp *"thorns in your side"* that serve as obstacles for you to overcome and grow stronger from.

The ancient rune þorn has many interpretations. For instance, it could signify strength and hardiness gained through harrowing experiences. Likewise, it foretells a warning of dangers and betrayal on the path ahead. However, some have theorized that its meaning *'thorn'* is a metaphor for Thor. He is the powerful half-giant son of Odin associated with thunder. This interpretation casts þorn as the rune of opposites and brute strength, reinforcing a complex and potent symbolism.

Þorn is a symbol and an example of wisdom from Norse mythology that can be applied to life today. Its relevance has endured through centuries, offering guidance for seekers who wish to grasp its symbolic and practical meanings.

Ōs (ᚩ)

"The mouth is the source of all language,
a pillar of wisdom and a comfort to wise men,
a blessing and a joy to every knight."
(Old English Rune Poem Verse 4)

The rune of truth and justice, ōs, has two different meanings in the futhorc. The first meaning is *'god,'* which refers to Odin specifically. This meaning mirrors ansuz (ᚨ) in the Elder Futhark and ós (ᚬ) in the Younger Futhark. Then, the second interpretation of ōs is as meaning *'mouth.'* Such interpretation is another reference to Odin, who has the *"breath of life,"* according to the Poetic Edda. Odin is also the master communicator able to inspire one and all. As such, ōs is the rune of the gods, inspiration, and communication with others and your higher self. Regarding our journey through the runic alphabet, ōs *(motivation and communication with the gods)* is the balance to þorn *(obstacles and the danger of demons)*. Similarly, this is the same as ós was to þhurs in the Younger Futhark and as ansuz is to thurisaz in the Elder Futhark.

When cast upright, ōs signifies that knowledge or communication with your higher self or other powers is incoming. As the rune of inspiration, ōs is a sign that divine energies are interested in you and your life's journey. Yet, if cast reversed, ōs is interpreted as a sign of miscommunication, misdirection through manipulation, or delusion about your goals or life's purpose.

Rād (R)

> *"Riding seems easy to every warrior while he is indoors*
> *and very courageous to him who traverses the high-roads*
> *on the back of a stout horse."*
> **(Old English Rune Poem Verse 5)**

Another rune that remains unchanged in the different runic scripts is rād (R). This rune is raidho (R) in the Elder Futhark and reið (R) in the Younger. Representing the journey, it sees us set out on our path of initiation into the greater mysteries of life and living. Cast upright, this rune is a sign that you are going through a time of personal evolution. It shows you are on the path to having the experiences you need to become the person you want to be. However, in merkstave, rād signifies you are becoming disconnected from your life's journey or purpose. Likewise, it tells that you must get back on track as soon as possible or risk facing unnecessary hardships.

Cēn (ᚳ)

"The torch is known to every living man by its pale, bright flame;
it always burns where princes sit within."
(Old English Rune Poem Verse 6)

Another place where the futhorc differs from the other two runic scripts is the inclusion of the *'c'* character of the alphabet. Where kaunan (ᚲ), meaning *'ulcer,'* represents the *'k'* sound alone. Then kaun (ᚴ), the Younger Futhark equivalent with the same meaning, represents the *'k,' 'g,'* and *'ŋ'* sounds, and cēn (ᚳ) stands for k and tʃ *(a strong 'ch' sound)*. Meaning *'torch,'* this is the rune of enlightenment. It represents the gaining of knowledge through learning and experience. Likewise, it means having the ability to improve our skill sets and begin to apply what we have learned back into the world.

Cēn, when cast upright, symbolizes gaining newfound knowledge and undergoing a process of personal development and growth. It is the essence of directed energy and indicates expertise in honing one's craft. On the other hand, if cēn appears reversed, it can reflect being out of sync with your inner guidance or having misplaced priorities. Additionally, reversed cēn may warn of an impersonal attitude, lack of awareness, or superiority complex.

Gyfu (X)

"Generosity brings credit and honor, which support one's dignity;
it furnishes help and subsistence
to all broken men who are devoid of aught else."
(Old English Rune Poem Verse 7)

While Freyr and Freyja's Ætt ends with kaun, the k-rune of the word futhark, the futhorc follows the ways of its parent script and includes two more runes in its first ætt. The first is gyfu (X), the evolution of gebo (X), which stands for *'gift.'* This is the rune of generosity and stands for equivalent exchange, in terms of what you put in is what you get out. As such, it is the 'gift' of improving yourself, enhancing your skills, and experiencing the world to the fullest.

When upright, gyfu shows that you are about to receive a *'gift'* of equivalent size to the sacrifice you have made to earn it. It can also mean that your vision is about to clear and that you have the divine blessing to continue. Yet, gyfu does not have a merkstave form. Nevertheless, if lying in opposition, it signifies over-dependence or greediness. Also, it is a sign of overly sacrificing oneself for no equivalent gain.

Wynn (ᚹ)

"Bliss, he enjoys who knows not suffering, sorrow nor anxiety, and has prosperity and happiness and a good enough house."
(Old English Rune Poem Verse 8)

The rune wynn (ᚹ) is one of the oldest runes in the futhorc, and its evolution from wunjo (ᚹ) is traced to the Elder Futhark alphabet. When read upright, this rune represents hope and harmony, symbolizing glory or spiritual rewards. Alternatively, if cast in merkstave, it is a sign of alienation, ignorance, and potential danger.

Throughout history, wynn has been associated with feelings of contentment stemming from correctly utilizing one's will or mastering a skill. It can also be interpreted as promoting accomplishment, prosperity, or fellowship. To further illustrate its significance, it may be helpful to mention that many Norse tribes would inscribe this rune on their weapons before heading into battle for protection from harm.

Heimdall's Ætt

Once the initiate has passed the tests and choices of Freyr or Freyja's Ætt, they receive the gift of wisdom and the reward earned for their sacrifices. When they realize this wisdom's glory and come to terms with their reward, the initiate is ready to move on to Heimdall's Ætt, the ætt of becoming a warrior.

Hægl (ᚺ)

> *"Hail is the whitest of grain;*
> *it is whirled from the vault of heaven*
> *and is tossed about by gusts of wind*
> *and then it melts into water."*
> **(Old English Rune Poem Verse 9)**

The rune 'hail' stands for life's unpredictable twists and turns. Think of it like preparing to move to a new city and encountering unexpected obstacles and opportunities. Turning to the rune shape, we see that it is a close copy of its parent rune, hagalaz (ᚺ), which was also drawn with a double-barred variant in some dialects of the Elder Futhark. Moreover, the h-rune of the Younger Futhark, hagall (*), looks quite different but carries the same meaning.

Hægl symbolizes the struggles needed to become resilient. As such, it is the rune of casting, tempering, testing, and enduring. Likewise, it is like forging a blade that requires constant patience and effort, and growing strong requires facing hardships and continuing. So, with the arrival of hægl, the first rune in Heimdall's Ætt, we are challenged to show our strength.

When hægl appears upright in your cast, it signifies growth and balance. However, it can also be an ominous sign pointing to danger or loss. For example, you could be preparing for a big move, and the rune warns you must prepare for any potential problems.

Nȳd (ᚾ)

"Trouble is oppressive to the heart;
yet often, it proves a source of help and salvation
to the children of men, to everyone who heeds it betimes."
(Old English Rune Poem Verse 10)

Next, we have nȳd, the futhorcian variant of naudiz and sibling to the Younger Futhark's nauðr. The runic shape (ᚾ), meaning *"need,"* and sound value (n) of this rune have remained the same since the Elder Futhark days. This is the rune of hardships and strength-building. It involves agreeing with Orlog (your destiny) and making it your own. While hægl pushes us with unexpected events, nȳd shapes us into our destined selves.

When cast upright, nȳd signifies an understanding of the fundamental truths of life. It is the drive of innovation and becoming more self-reliant. Conversely, it can be a warning of lack or difficulty when it appears reversed. For instance, if you want to achieve your dream career but keep finding nȳd in your readings, it may indicate that you need to reassess your plan and make some changes to get closer to your goal.

Īs (ᛁ)

"Ice is very cold and immeasurably slippery;
it glistens as clear as glass and is most like to gem;
it is a floor wrought by the frost, fair to look upon."
(Old English Rune Poem Verse 11)

Another rune that has not changed much in the main runic alphabets is the i-rune of isaz from the Elder Futhark, íss from the

Younger Futhark, and īs from the futhorc. All three mean *'ice'* and represent the rune of self-control and focus. On our runic journey, īs symbolizes the stillness and fortitude of mind we must develop to keep our egos in check. After the tempering and molding the last two runes, īs deals with cooling and solidifying. As we gain more spiritual knowledge and greater spiritual awareness through the tests and trials we face and overcome, we become more headstrong. As such, our egos will inevitably grow to match our new strengths. Īs serves as a reminder to develop the self-control and the stillness of mind necessary to keep this strengthening ego in check.

When cast upright, īs is a sign of growing clarity or developing self-awareness. With no merkstave form, it indicates self-aggrandizement, egoistic behavior, over-indulgence, or other forms of losing self-control.

Gēr (ᛡ)

"Summer is a joy to men when God, the holy King of Heaven, suffers the earth to bring forth shining fruits for rich and poor alike."
(Old English Rune Poem Verse 12)

The Anglo-Saxon symbol of jēran (ᛄ), otherwise known as the j-rune from the Elder Futhark, is also known as gēr (ᛡ). This rune has a double meaning, with both interpretations being *'good harvest'* or *'good year.'* Cast upright, gēr represents an acknowledgment for all the hard work and positive actions undertaken. It suggests that reaping the rewards of your journey is just around the corner. Additionally, it stands tall as a sign of peace and prosperity.

Unfortunately, being cast in opposition can signify poor timing, stagnation, and regression. Gēr does not have a merkstave form, which could represent an inability to progress due to inconvenient timing opportunities. It comprises two parts; a spearhead pointing upwards to embody success and an arrow pointing downward to characterize a lack of momentum.

Ēoh (ᛇ)

> *"The yew is a tree with rough bark,*
> *hard and fast in the earth, supported by its roots,*
> *a guardian of flame and a joy upon an estate."*
> **(Old English Rune Poem Verse 13)**

The representation of Yggdrasil in the runic alphabet, ēoh (ᛇ), is the evolution of eihwaz (ᛇ) from the Elder Futhark. This is a rune that was cut from the Younger Futhark. Meaning *'yew tree,'* ēoh is the rune of life, death, and renewal. It is the rune of the world tree, the tree of life. By life and death, ēoh does not only means the coming and leaving from this mortal coil. Yet, it signifies the life of new habits or the end of unwanted personality traits. In our journey through the runic alphabet, ēoh represents the growth of the individual over the years. Like a tree sheds its leaves in the winter before growing new ones in the spring, we leave parts of ourselves behind and develop new skills as we continue down the path of life.

If cast upright, ēoh foretells making moves toward achieving enlightenment or that you are on the right path to obtaining what you seek. But cast merkstave is a sign of dissatisfaction, weakness, or confusion.

Peorð (ᛈ)

> *"Peorth is a source of recreation and amusement to the great,*
> *where warriors sit blithely together in the banqueting hall."*
> **(Old English Rune Poem Verse 14)**

The p-rune of the Futhorc is Peorð (ᛈ), which evolved from its precursor, perthro (ᛈ), a rune that does not appear in the

Younger Futhark. As such, its closest modern English translation is an equivalent phrase for *'lot cup,'* used by Vikings to play a game of fate. This special rune encompasses the potential, chances, and luck that each person experiences on their life journey. If peorð appears right side up, it forecasts good fortune and success. However, when reversed, it signals hardships beyond our control.

Eolh (ᛉ)

> *"The eolh-sedge is mostly to be found in a marsh;*
> *it grows in the water and makes a ghastly wound,*
> *covering with blood every warrior who touches it."*
> **(Old English Rune Poem Verse 15)**

After the peorð rune comes the x-rune of the futhorc, eolh (ᛉ). This symbol carries a deeply spiritual and protective meaning. It is the Anglo-Saxon equivalent of the Elder Futhark's z-rune, algiz (ᛉ), while its younger counterpart is the R-rune, yr (ᛦ). These three runes have different names and meanings: algiz and eolh being 'elk,' while yr translates to *'yew.'* While this rune can be seen as a sign of death in the Younger Futhark, it signifies rebirth and protection in Elder and Anglo-Saxon runic scripts.

The deeper spiritual significance behind casting eolh includes the growth of personal strength and protection from danger. When cast upright, it indicates a blooming connection with your higher self by allowing yourself to be open to messages from above. However, the reverse side of this same rune portrays separation from this connection or danger that may arise on your path. As such, it may suggest caution rather than joyous celebration during its interpretation.

Sigel (ᛋ)

> *"The sun is ever a joy in the hopes of seafarers
> when they journey away over the fish's bath,
> until the courser of the deep bears them to land."*
> **(Old English Rune Poem Verse 16)**

The final rune of Heimdall's Ætt, the ætt of the warrior, is sigel (ᛋ). Meaning *'sun,'* this is the evolution of sowilō (ᛊ) from the Elder Futhark and sibling to sól (ᛋ) from the Younger Futhark. All carry the same meaning, with sigel and sól identical in their runic shape. Sigel is the rune of success. Like Freyr and Freyja's Ætt ends positively with gyfu *(gift)* and wynn *(joy or bliss)*, so does Heimdall's. With eolh, we connect to the divine and with our higher selves. With sigel, we reach the success and wholeness that comes from achieving victory in battle or mastery of a skill.

Sigel appearing upright in your casting is a sign of guidance or hope. It signifies that you are on track to achieving your goals and are living your life's purpose. However, sigel does not have a merkstave form. Lying in opposition means false success, bad advice, or losing sight of your goals or purpose.

Týr's Ætt

Týr, the God of Justice and heroic patron, presides over the final ætt of the runic alphabet. This ætt is associated with being a skilled warrior, embodying all the necessary traits to excel in their chosen field. Unlike Heimdall's Ætt, which covers trials and tests to become a warrior, this is the stage where one becomes one, completing the third stage of life and our journey through rune lore. This stage marks an initiation into understanding divinity and its profound meanings.

Tīr (↑)

> *"Tiw is a guiding star; well, does it keep faith with princes;*
> *it is ever on its course over the mists of night and never fails."*
> **(Old English Rune Poem Verse 17)**

The first rune in the futhork's third ætt is tīr (↑), the evolution of tiwaz (↑) from the Elder Futhark, with its sister being týr (↑). All three refer to the enigmatic god of the Germanic peoples, Tyr. This is the rune of justice and sacrifice. In the Anglo-Saxon Rune Poem, tīr represents the *"guiding star"* (North Star). Used by sailors in ancient times to navigate the seas in the northern hemisphere, this star came to symbolize a moral compass and a physical one. A spark of order and control in the cosmos, Tyr is the god of order, control, and justice. On our runic journey, tīr represents the building of our willpower and developing our moral compasses as we become spiritually awakened humans.

Cast upright, tīr is a sign of honesty, justice, and victory achieved through faith in the divine, loyalty to your moral compass, or self-sacrifice. The merkstave of tīr warns of mental paralysis, over-analyzing, or overly sacrificing yourself. It can also indicate injustice or some other kind of imbalance.

Beorc (ᛒ)

> *"The poplar bears no fruit; yet without seed, it brings forth suckers,*
> *for it is generated from its leaves.*
> *Splendid are its branches and gloriously adorned*
> *its lofty crown which reaches to the skies."*
> **(Old English Rune Poem Verse 18)**

Beorc is another rune that mostly stays the same between the different runic alphabets. The runic shape (ᛒ), meaning (birch), and sound value [b] remain the same in all three, except the

Younger Futhark adds the *'p'* sound to its version of ᛒ, björk. In the Elder Futhark, it goes by the name *'berkanen.'* This is the rune of the Birch Goddess, birth, and sanctuary. As the first tree to come back to life as winter changes to spring, the birch symbolizes the cycle of life*: birth, death, and rebirth.* With ēoh, this cycle is not just about the birth or death of a person. Yet, more to do with the birth, death, and rebirth that happens as the seasons change and we grow into different versions of ourselves. Likewise, Beorc is the rune of female fertility and the fruition of ideas and goals.

In its upright position is a sign of becoming, a changing lifestyle, or sanctuary through divine protection and healing. Although it cannot be cast merkstave, beorc is a sign of sterility, stagnation, blurred vision, or conspiring forces when lying in opposition.

Eh (ᛖ)

> *"The horse is a joy to princes in the presence of warriors.*
> *A steed in the pride of its hoofs*
> *when rich men on horseback bandy words about it;*
> *and it is ever a source of comfort to the restless."*
> **(Old English Rune Poem Verse 19)**

Next is the e-rune of the futhorc and the evolution of ehwaz (ᛖ) from the Elder Futhark, eh (ᛖ). This rune does not appear in the Younger Futhark. Meaning *'horse,'* eh is the rune of travel and progress. It symbolizes the outer and inner journeys we take in life and the trust we must have in the *'vehicle'* or *'steed'* that is our body. Like a horse with a skilled rider, eh represents the symbiotic relationship we must have with ourselves and others.

If cast upright, eh signifies harmony, loyalty, or friendship. It can also be a sign of collaboration and trust. In merkstave form, eh is a sign of disharmony, betrayal, or an enemy acting against you. Finally, it can also indicate indecisiveness or mistrust of your path.

Mann (ᛗ)

> *"The joyous man is dear to his kinsmen;*
> *yet every man is doomed to fail his fellow,*
> *since the Lord, by his decree, will commit the vile*
> *carrion to the earth."*
> **(Old English Rune Poem Verse 20)**

With the meaning of 'man' or 'humankind,' mann is a rune that embodies intelligence, planning, and increased awareness. It is featured in the Elder Futhark and Younger Futhark runes, mannaz (ᛗ) in the former and maðr (ᛘ) in the latter. When we progress on our runic journey, mann symbolizes our ambition to reach out for self-discovery, to be closer to what resides inside us. This rune also speaks of humanity's capability to shape reality with otherworldly forces and natural elements.

Having it cast upright, mann carries energies invigorating intelligence and awakened understanding and realization of one's inner potential. In contrast, when presented in merkstave mode, it may induce depressive states or unrealistic feelings of superiority, a manifestation of mortals' emotional hurdles.

Lagu (ᛚ)

> *"The ocean seems interminable to men,*
> *if they venture on the rolling bark*
> *and the waves of the sea terrify them*
> *and the courser of the deep heed, not its bridle."*
> **(Old English Rune Poem Verse 21)**

The rune lagu is believed to be one of the oldest runes in practice. It originates from the Proto-Germanic language and has been used in different runic alphabets for centuries. Although it keeps a similar shape and sound, the interpretations vary slightly between cultures.

From the Elder Futhark, laguz refers to *'lake,'* while in Younger Futhark, it could symbolize *'water'* or *'waterfall.'* In the Anglo-Frissian period, lagu was known as the *'ocean'* or *'sea.'* Moreover, it stands for life energy and intuition powering any evolutionary process.

In divination, this rune gave a positive connotation when appearing upright: *passing tests and achieving growth.* On the other hand, its reversed position could indicate that someone might be lost in fantasies or controlled by manipulative forces.

Ing (ᛝ)

> *"Ing was first seen by men among the East Danes,*
> *till followed by his chariot,*
> *he departed eastwards over the waves.*
> *So, the Heardingas named the hero."*
> **(Old English Rune Poem Verse 22)**

The ŋ-rune of the futhorc, ing (ᛝ), is found in the Elder Futhark as inguz (◊) but is not included in the Younger Futhark. Ing's shape changed from the parent alphabet to the child, but the meaning remained. They represent the Proto-Germanic god Ing or Inwi. This god was known as Yngvi in Old Norse and Ingþine in Old English and is an earlier name for Freyr.

Before he became known by the moniker 'Lord,' Freyr was known as Ing. Freyr is the god of fertility, peace, and good weather. As such, ing is associated with the meaning *'seed.'* This is the rune of earth, agriculture, male fertility, and sexuality. On our runic journey, ing represents the act or process of creation. The best way to think of this rune is like the way we use the suffix -ing at the end of verbs to add action to it. Doing, being, creating; the process of activity and creation.

When cast upright, ing is a sign of gestation, growth, or spending time to improve oneself. Ing cannot be reversed, but lying in opposition is a sign of frivolous behavior, immaturity, taking action, or putting in effort without gaining positive change.

Ēðel (ᛟ)

> *"An estate is very dear to every man,*
> *if he can enjoy there in his house*
> *whatever is right and proper in constant prosperity."*
> **(Old English Rune Poem Verse 23)**

With the meaning of *'heritage'* or *'inheritance,'* ēðel (ᛟ) is the futhorc's version of the o-rune from the Elder Futhark, othala (ᛟ). This is the rune of home, connecting with your ancestors and drawing on and adding to the spiritual power from your ancestral land. Ēðel provides a link to the rune feoh (wealth), the first letter of the runic alphabet.

In the Elder Futhark, othala is the 24th and final rune that symbolizes inheritance, home, and land. Meanwhile, in the Younger Futhark, it is moved to become second last. This switch in position suggests the importance of taking a moment to reflect on how you use your wealth before embarking on a journey to come full circle. Furthermore, this spiritual journey is only possible when understanding the meaning behind each rune and how each relates to one other. Such knowledge can help us expand our understanding of our past, present, and future and live consciously as part of a greater cycle.

Upright, ēðel means prosperity, freedom, and the betterment of your group. Reversed, ēðel speaks of poverty, homelessness, or losing touch with one's ancestral land. Likewise, it is a sign of mistreatment, such as racism or xenophobia.

Dæg (ᛞ)

"Day, the glorious light of the Creator, is sent by the Lord;
it is beloved of men, a source of hope and happiness
for the rich and poor,
and of service to all."
(Old English Rune Poem Verse 24)

For the final runic symbol of Týr's Ætt, the futhorc rune dæg (ᛞ) is derived from the Elder Futhark's dagaz (ᛞ). Both runes hold a similar meaning of *'day'* or *'dawn'* and share the same shape. It marks the end of a journey depicting the life and purpose of human life. Likewise, it represents the unity of one's self, synthesis with the environment, and connecting opposites to gain enlightenment.

When cast upright, dæg symbolizes an awakening, alertness, or an upcoming positive shift. On the contrary, if it lies in opposition, then it means someone is blind to their predicament or that an unfavorable situation is likely to arise. This highlights how important it is for people to consider their pasts and futures, living in the moment while being aware of what may come next.

Other Runes

Although the journey may be over for the three ættir of the runic script, this is not the end of the futhorc's extended alphabet. There are still five more runes in the Anglo-Saxon rune poem, totaling 29. In some dialects of the futhorc, it was then further extended by four more runes to reach a total of 33 characters in its runic alphabet. The futhorc can be used either in its 24 runes version derived from the Elder Futhark or in its 26-rune version where āc (ᚪ), 'oak,' and æsc (ᚫ), 'ash' are included. Along with ōs (ᚩ), 'god,' these runes are the evolution of the a-rune from the Elder Futhark. Ansuz (ᚨ), split into three different sounds, accommodates Old English's developing vowels and other Anglo-Frissian languages. After that comes the runes that were added later, as Old English and the futhorc developed, and have no connection to the runes of the Elder Futhark. Let us go through these final runes of the Anglo-Saxon futhorc.

Āc (ᚪ)

> *"The oak fattens the flesh of pigs for the children of men.*
> *Often it traverses the gannet's bath,*
> *and the ocean proves whether the oak keeps faith*
> *in an honorable fashion."*
> **(Old English Rune Poem Verse 25)**

Āc, one of the runes of Elder Futhark, is derived from its parent rune ansuz (ᚨ), which translates to 'god.' This symbolizes the potential for small beginnings to blossom into something greater with continuous growth and progress. Represented by an acorn growing into a mighty oak tree, it reflects the power of potentiality. It stands for strength and endurance, used to build ships due to its incredible ability to withstand storms and strong winds.

When cast upright, āc indicates that you have all the resources required to succeed; if these are not present, they shall soon be acquired. There is also an indication of making good use of one's potential. Conversely, when cast merkstave, it speaks of a hindering obstacle that could threaten your growth and warns against not utilizing one's potential fully.

Æsc (ᚫ)

> *"The ash is exceedingly high and precious to men.
> With its sturdy trunk, it offers a stubborn resistance,
> though attacked by many a man."*
> **(Old English Rune Poem Verse 26)**

The third child of ansuz (ᚫ) is the æ-rune, æsc (ᚫ), from the futhorc. This runic symbol is closely related to the ash tree. Like its elder sibling, the oak is a dependable and vitally important resource for weapon manufacture and crafting. Instilled with stability and resilience in times of hardship, upright æsc serves as a beacon of protection, hope, and healing for those who bear it. Conversely, when reversed, this rune denotes a period of difficulty where one may feel overpowered by external stubbornness or other obstacles.

With this symbolism, there are plenty more fascinating facts surrounding ash trees and their uses throughout history. Not only have they been integral to Norse mythology as sacred places of worship. Yet, they have also been used to create tools such as mallets and axes since ancient times. Furthermore, both their wood and bark were integral components in various medications due to the antiseptic properties discovered in them. Altogether these qualities make the runes associated with the ash tree some of the most reliable symbols for safety and security, according to Futharks lore.

Ȳr (ᚣ)

*"Yr is a source of joy and honor to every prince and knight;
it looks well on a horse and is reliable equipment for a journey."*
(Old English Rune Poem Verse 27)

Associated with the yew tree, the y-rune of mastery, ȳr (ᚣ), is the second rune in the Futhorc. This symbolizes the longbow, an iconic and powerful weapon used throughout history. It calls for dedication to art, sport, or any skill you master. Furthermore, if upright, it promises capability and potential success in what you set out to do. However, if reversed, it warns against a lack of required skills, laziness, or inertia hindering progress.

To use this power effectively, one must understand its deep cultural roots. According to Norse mythology, the first longbow was created by Ullr (Oller), a skilled master archer who lived alongside Odin in Asgard. Before his death, he also tutored his beloved son Baldr using bows and arrows. This connection between Ullr and ȳr brings a reverence for a craft that has been central throughout time.

Ior (ᛡ)

*"Iar is a river fish, and yet it always feeds on land;
it has a fair abode encompassed by water, where
it lives in happiness."*
Old English Rune Poem Verse 28)

Ior (ᛡ) is the io-rune (yo) of the futhorc carrying the meaning of *'eel.'* This is a variant of the j-rune, gēr (ᛄ), which means *'year'* or *'harvest.'* Ior, on the other hand, represents Jörmungandr, the World Serpent. Along with Fenrir and Hel, Jörmungandr is a child of Loki and the giantess Angrboða, who were all foretold to be the ones to bring about Ragnarök. As such, the three children were separated; Hel was sent to the underworld, Fenrir remained under watch in Asgard, and Jörmungandr, the middle child, was thrown into the oceans of Midgard (Earth). In the depths of the oceans, the World Serpent grew to encircle the globe and then bit down on its tail, representing the ouroboros. When Jörmungandr releases its tail once more, Ragnarök will commence.

As such, ior is a protective or binding rune. More than that, this rune represents a snake. As a serpent can live both in water and on land, this is the rune of the duality of life. When ior appears upright, it signifies the death of something old, the birth of something new, or a combination of both. However, ior cannot be cast merkstave, but when in opposition, unavoidable hardships or danger are coming up.

Ēar (ᛠ)

> *"The grave is horrible to every knight,*
> *when the corpse quickly begins to cool*
> *and is laid in the bosom of the dark earth.*
> *Prosperity declines and happiness passes away*
> *and covenants are broken."*
> **(Old English Rune Poem Verse 29)**

The last character in the Anglo-Saxon Rune Poem is ēar (ᛠ), the ea-rune of the futhorc. With the meaning of *'grave,'* this is the rune of the past, ending, or death. This rune was a late addition to the futhorc, with its first use recorded in the 9th century. While other runes dealing with death did so in a way that captured the growth that occurs through the ending of one thing and the beginning of another, ēar is death personified or symbolized. Upright, ēar speaks of a happy ending or the completion of some goal or task. Merkstave, ēar is an omen of death or loss and sadness.

Northumbrian Runes

Rune diviners and enthusiasts discovered the Northumbrian Runes in the 8th century AD as an addition to the Anglo-Saxon futhorc. Some individuals have adopted these runes to supplement their divination practices, providing a more comprehensive range of symbols. The interpretation of these four characters can be personalized for the individual user based on what resonates with them naturally. Although the Latin script replaced the futhorc for Old English writing, these runes can still be used to benefit from their full potential in spells and other forms of magick.

Cweorð (ᛢ)

As an iconic symbol of transformation in the Anglo-Saxon rune, cweorð or cpeorð (ᛢ) reflects the use of flames in a myriad of ways. As such, it is a source of heat and light, a method to purify the deceased and their souls, or an emblem of strength. It has roots in peorð (ᛈ), the p-rune of the futhorc. In addition, it is the second fire rune in the futhorc, preceded by cēn (ᚳ), which denotes 'torch' and stands for enlightenment.

When upright, this rune stands for courage and endurance in overcoming life's challenges, with transformation being its primary connotation. On the other hand, if it appears reversed, it signals potential destructive forces at work that may prevent you from achieving your goal. Its associated meanings can be further contextualized through a closer look at how the fire was viewed by Anglo-Saxons, providing them with security and sanctity in their homes and offering liberation during funeral pyres.

Calc (ᛣ)

The next Northumbrian rune is calc, another form of k-rune that means *'chalice'* (calic) or *'chalk'* (cealc). What calc refers to is unknown, but the 'chalice' definition fits better for divination purposes. Under this meaning, 'calc' refers to a ritual cup or goblet and invokes the legend of the Holy Grail from the tales of King Arthur and the Knights of Camelot. Calc is the rune of offerings, as a chalice is used to drink from during a ceremony. It also symbolizes the death and rebirth that an individual goes through during a ceremony and the natural ending of things that inevitably must happen. When cast upright, calc is a sign of something coming to a positive conclusion or an upcoming spiritual transformation. Then, if cast merkstave, calc warns of an untimely termination of something or an unexpected sacrifice.

Stan (ᛥ)

With the meaning of *'stone'* and the sound value of *'st,'* stan symbolizes not only the immovable obstruction that stone can be. Yet, it can also be the little game pieces made of stone. Stan is the rune of material obstacles and the unavoidable difficulties we face. It also symbolizes the link between our divine souls and earthly bodies. Stan appearing upright signifies strength, achievement, and the skill and ability to overcome obstructions in your path. Meanwhile, stan does not have a merkstave form but means a blockage, obstacle, or other upcoming hardships and difficulties.

Gar (ᚸ)

The futhorc is an alphabet of 33 runes believed to possess immense power, covering three pillars of runology: Runic Scripts, Casting, and Divination. Gar, or $\bar{g}$, is the final rune in the extended Anglo-Saxon futhorc. It symbolizes success in battle and carries the meaning of *'spear,'* a reference to Odin's Gungnir, which never missed its target. In terms of sound, it is similar to gyfu (gift), but a victory from gar comes from more hard work than from receiving a gift. When upright, it represents a reward for hard work or suspicion of success. However, lying in opposition can be interpreted as a loss or hindrance to achieving your goals.

Pillar 3
Casting

Now is the time to take your understanding of runes and the varying runic scripts to the next level by divining your future. The Elder Futhark, Viking runes from the Younger Futhark, and Old English from the Anglo-Saxon futhorc, each of these runic alphabets offers something different. Before you begin casting, consider which best resonates with your inner self, as it can become a powerful vehicle for exploring your fate.

Unlocking a deeper understanding of runology will give you all you need to interpret and synthesize information through rune casting. Visualization, meditation, and reflection create an environment conducive to exploring higher knowledge. This allows us to connect deeply with symbolism and its meaning, uncovering our destinies.

6

What You Need to Know About Rune Casting

Rune casting has helped to guide people through life and all its big decisions since before. The runes were formed into the alphabet known as the Elder Futhark. This makes divination and magic the original uses of the runes. Their use as a writing system comes in a distant second. As with reading Tarot cards, casting runes is not a form of fortune telling or some ineffable way of predicting the future. Instead, the runes provide insights into specific questions that you ask. They do this by delivering our influential subconscious minds with a potent medium to solve the *'problem'* of the question asked. Our brains are massive problem-solving machines; all they need is the right key to unlock the true potential of the human mind. The runes were initially recorded by Odin the Allfather as he sought to understand the mysteries of life and the cosmos. For instance, they are the perfect key for unlocking the divine within us all, guiding you to the answer you seek, but your higher self already knows.

In this chapter, we will talk about everything rune casting, from the history of rune casting, to how to make your own rune sets, before ending with how to cast runes.

History of Rune Casting

By the nature of runes, mystery and secrecy surround their earliest use. The word *'rune'* means *'secret message,'* after all. Rock carvings found in Northern Europe and throughout Scandinavia from the Bronze and early Iron Ages are believed to be the earliest incarnation of runic writing. As we said in Chapter 1, the first mention of the runes being used for divination and magical purposes is from *Germania 10,* written by the Roman historian Tacitus in the 1st century AD. Tacitus describes the classical way of making runes (cutting a branch from a nut-bearing tree and slicing it into strips before carving runes on each) and casting them.

As the prolific historian explains, the runes were randomly thrown onto a white cloth, as you would shuffle the Tarot deck before laying out the cards. Then, a priest or the family's father would say a prayer to the gods in which they would invoke the blessings of specific deities. After doing so, they would then ask their question and, staring up at the heavens, move their hand over the cast as they pick the first of three runes. After being drawn to a specific rune, the caster would pick it up and interpret it in terms of the meaning of the rune and how it was positioned compared to the caster (upright, merkstave, or lying in opposition). Once the first rune has been selected and interpreted, the caster repeats the process for the remaining two runes of the cast, analyzing each as they are chosen before giving an overall divination for the three runes cast and how they relate to the question asked.

And so finishes Tacitus' historical account of the use of runes for divination. Interestingly, while this account comes from the first century, it is only around the fourth century AD that the alphabet known as the Elder Futhark became commonly used throughout Scandinavia and northern Europe.

How to Cast Runes

Now that we know more about the history of rune casting, it is time to turn to the runes themselves. This section will cover how to make your own rune sets and what materials to make them from. After that, we will dive deeper into the world of rune casting and how you can best draw on the magic and divine energies of these ancient and timeless symbols to enhance your daily life.

Making Your Own Rune Set

The first thing you will need after knowledge to cast runes is the rune set itself. You can buy a set of runes; there is nothing wrong with doing so. Search " *rune sets*" on your chosen browser or Amazon, and you will get a miasma of great options for masterful craftsmanship. Make sure to read the customer reviews before selecting one, and you are onto a winner of having your rune set in no time. If you are wondering whether you should buy a wood, stone, metal, glass, or crystal rune set, we will get to that next up in this section.

For the more crafty people who prefer the hands-on approach of making their own rune sets, let us go through the steps you will need to follow and the things you need to know to do so.

1. Choose Your Materials

As we saw in Tacitus' account, the primary material used to make a rune set in ancient times was wood, preferably from a nut-bearing tree, but this is not the only option out there, and you are more than free to choose a different one if it resonates with your energy more. In fact, this is crucial. Here are the most commonly used materials that runes are made out of:

Wood

The favored material for making runes throughout history has been wood. As we saw in the breakdown of the rune meanings, some runes directly symbolize trees. Trees were an integral part of Norse mythology, with the runes appearing to Odin on the bark of Yggdrasil, the world tree. Yggdrasil is considered an ash tree, so this is often the wood chosen for making runes. However, any nut or seed (fruit) bearing tree will serve fine. You could use yew, birch, or oak, for example. Before cutting the branch off your chosen tree, ask permission beforehand to ensure the right energy is stored in the wood you will use to make your runes. Also, leave an offering of water for the tree after chopping off the branch to complete the ceremony.

If you want to make your runes out of wood but do not have access to the right kind of trees or do not want to cut them, you can buy blank wooden rune sets online. Once you have your slices or blocks of wood, then comes the time to either paint, carve, or pyrograph (burn into the wood) the runes onto them, but more on this later.

Pebbles or Stones

If you live near a beach, river, or mountain, you could create your rune set out of the pebbles or small stones you collect from there. It is not just about the power of the runic symbols but also the energy you put into them that matters, and connecting your rune set to the land you live in is always a great idea. Remember that engraving runes in stone is much harder than carving them on wood. You could opt to paint your pebble rune set, but this will fade over time unless properly cared for.

Bones

A more controversial material to use for your rune set is bone. Some people enjoy the more shamanistic image of casting bones, and since it is all about the energy you put into making and using them, there is nothing wrong with that. Just try to ensure that the bones come from an animal that died of natural causes or, if hunted, a similar prayer and offers were made to honor the animal's sacrifice as would be made for cutting a branch from a tree.

Clay

From the macabre to the mundane, clay is our final common material to make your rune set. Clay is easy to work with and easy to engrave runes on. Just make sure to bake and seal your clay runes properly to ensure they remain chip-free for as long as possible.

Whichever material you use to make your rune set, the key is consistency in size and shape. Also, ensure your runes are small enough to cast in your hands. Once you have chosen your material and have a strip of wood, pebble, or clay piece ready for each rune, the time to begin creating a rune set comes.

2. Begin the Ritual

First, you will need to select a sacred space or a place where you feel most comfortable and have room to work. If you have not sanctified a place in your house for such things before, you can perform the Hammer Rite or Hammarsetning to do so. This space protection rite draws on Mjolnir, Thor's hammer's power to protect and consecrate a specific area around you. Thor is the protector of Asgard and Midgard; with his mighty hammer, he separates order and chaos. To perform the Hammer Rite, stand up straight in your workspace and visualize yourself holding Mjolnir out. Invoke Thor's name in sanctifying and protecting your space as you hold Mjolnir in the four cardinal directions, beginning with the north. Then, hold the hammer up to the sky above you before facing it below you to complete the sphere of protection. Once this is done, your space is ready to begin working on your runes.

Think over the mystical history of the runes and invite the gods or goddesses who rule over them into your space as you consecrate it for the inscription of your runes. Odin, Freyja and Freyr, Heimdall, and Týr; invite these deities to add their energies to the creation of your rune set. Pour a symbolic tot of wine, apple juice, or milk for the gods as you ask them to steady and guide your hand in the task. Invoke the blessings of your ancestors and invite any other wights (spirits or supernatural beings) you feel connected to or wish to have around. With your materials laid out in front of you, dedicate this moment to the creation of runes, and when you are ready, pick up your first strip, tablet, or pebble, and call on Freyja and Freyr as you inscribe the runes of their ætt.

Say the rune out loud once you are done painting or carving it, and remind yourself of its meaning and interpretations as you do so. Hold the rune up to your mouth as you name it, visualizing what most reminds you of that specific rune. Let us take fehu, for example. Visualize what you most strongly associate with *'wealth,'* concentrate on this as you carve or paint, and imbue the rune with this energy, as you name it. Once you inscribe the rune, place it on a white cloth or napkin.

Traditionally, runes would also be made yours completely by tracing the runic symbol with your blood. This stains the runes with your unique *"fluid of life."* This is by no means compulsory. If you stain your runes, you could mix a few drops of blood into red paint or prick your finger and trace the lines. As for the paint, you could use red acrylic paint, or a mixture of red ochre and linseed oil works just as well.

3. Consecrate Your Rune Set

After allowing your runes to dry, sit back down and re-invite the gods into your space. Meditate for a bit on the purpose of the runes and their powerful potential to help you achieve what you seek. Concentrate on the magical nature of the runes, ruminate on the magic that exists all around us just beyond sight. Accept the divine gift of these symbols that allow us to comprehend the mysteries of the cosmos through runology. Then, if you have not done so already, arrange your runes in order and separate them into the ættir so that you have three rows of eight runes each on your white casting cloth.

Go through each rune once more, tracing the symbol with your eyes, visualizing that which you most associate with its esoteric meaning as you name it. Take your time to intensely focus on each rune in your set, thinking over the runic journey we discussed in the previous paragraph as you do so. Then, when you are done, thank the gods, goddesses, ancestors, and wights for their participation in the creation of the runes. Your runes are now sealed and ready for use!

Using Your Runes

With your freshly made or bought rune set, you can begin casting and reading these timeless signs of cosmic forces. In other words, it is time to learn about the process of rune casting.

Prepare Your Space

One thing that will get you in the right headspace for casting runes is to begin each time in the same way and place. This ritual could include placing your runes out in front of you on a white cloth before meditating on them for a while. You could also light candles or set out crystals to help create the right ambiance or vibe. After that, ensure that you are facing north and get comfortable. Then, invite the gods and ask them for their blessing and energy in the reading to come. If you are in a new place, conduct the Hammer Rite to sanctify the space before laying out your runes.

Form Your Question

To tap into the runes' divine powers, you need to have a specific question to ask them. Think carefully about what you seek to ask and how best to word it. *"Yes-No"* questions do not work for rune casting, so express your question in a more general, open-ended way. Rather than *"Will I get this job?"* you could say, *"What are the chances that I will get this job?"* for example. Or, better yet, *"How will it feel once I have this job?"* You must focus on your feelings behind the question and use this energy to guide your reading.

Cast the Runes

With your question in mind, pick up your runes and shake them in your hands. Hold them up to your lips as you speak your question before casting them out onto your casting cloth. The best way for beginners to go from here is to remove all the runes that fell face-down and set them aside. Then, gather the remaining runes, repeat your question, and cast them out again. Remove any face-down runes and continue this until you have five or fewer left in the cast. Once you do, leave these runes as they fall on your casting cloth.

Read their Meaning

With five or fewer runes remaining, it is time to read their meanings. It is best to write down the runes and their positions in a journal before interpreting how they answer your question. Record the runes from left to right. Also, note if the rune was cast upright, merkstave (upside down), or in opposition (sideways). Then, work on divining what these specific runes and their position mean for you and your question. Refer to the earlier chapters of this book as and when you need to review how to interpret the different runes.

Tools of the Trade

Now that we know how to make our runes and the basics of rune casting, it is time to go over the different tools of the trade for runology. These are the things, besides this book and your rune set, that you will want to get to enhance your casting and make divining simpler and more efficient.

Rune Pouch

The first thing you want to get to protect your runes is a rune pouch. This is the bag you keep your runes in to keep them from getting damaged or lost and to make them easily transportable for when you are doing your rune casting on the move. If you prefer a wooden box or another container to keep your runes in, that is perfectly fine, too. Whatever you choose, pick something that aesthetically represents and protects your rune set.

Casting Cloth

As mentioned earlier in this chapter, we cast runes onto a white cloth called a 'casting cloth.' This is done to keep the runes from getting scuffed or damaged, as well as to enhance the energy of the reading. A casting cloth, called a *'rune cloth' or 'altar cloth,'* can be as plain or patterned as you want it to be. It can be as large or small as you like. Make sure you can cast all your runes onto it comfortably. It can also be any most appealing shape, with round and square being the usual choices. You could make your rune cloth or buy one online. Some people choose to have protective runes patterned on their casting cloth, while others prefer to use it as a *'map'* that serves as another layer to their readings. This is used for more advanced casting methods, as seen in Chapter 7.

The *'map'* of a rune cloth generally comprises a central circle encompassed by a larger circle divided into four sections. Then, four lines connect the outer circle to the four corners of your casting cloth. This design symbolizes the nine worlds. Midgard (Earth) in the central circle, with Asgard in the North-East quadrant of the outer circle. Below Asgard is Svartalfheim (the realm of the dark elves or dwarves), with Hel to the left of it. Making up the final of the four is Álfheim (the realm of the light elves). The outer North area belongs to Muspelheim (the realm of fire), the East to Vanaheimr (the realm of the Vanir), the South to Niflheim (the realm of ice), and Jötunheimr (the realm of the first giants). This makes up the nine realms of Norse mythology.

Casting Pillow

Known as a 'stol,' this is a pillow embroidered or painted with runes you sit on while casting runes. This is to increase your comfort (especially when casting outdoors) and call upon the rune's energies on your stol when casting. Sitting on a casting pillow also means you are raised a little higher above your casting cloth, allowing you to reign over your runes like a god looking down at another plane.

Mearmots

Mearmots are personal talismans or magical items that you use to focus your mind and add to the energy of the casting. These could include candles, crystals, precious stones, or other objects that get you in the zone for reading runes. Besides the talismans that you bring to each casting, you should also try to bring something with you related to the question you are going to be asking of the runes. For example, if you are asking a question related to someone in your family, bring a picture of them or something that belongs to them. If you are doing a casting for someone else, then ask them to bring along mearmots that are special to them and are related to the question they plan to ask of the runes.

Pen, Pencil, and Paper

The final tools you need for your rune castings are a pen or pencil and a journal to record yours. While it is not essential to write down your readings, it is beneficial, as new interpretations can arise as you write them down. Keeping a rune journal lets, you easily notice patterns and trends in your readings. It is also useful to keep a summary of the rune meanings written down at the front of your rune journal. Finally, it is also a good idea to write down your question before you begin the casting to cement it in your mind and help you focus on it.

With the tools of the runic trade, we have finished with another chapter and another pillar of runology! You are now ready to put the runes to use. We covered a basic casting method in this chapter, but in the next, we will go over some different kinds of runic spreads and more advanced layouts as we move onto the fourth pillar of Runology: Spreads and Layouts.

Pillar 4
Layouts and Spreads

With all the background knowledge you need to become a pro rune caster, you are ready to start using the runes. The first three pillars provided us with the foundational understanding of Runology. Now, it is time to put all that knowledge to use and start casting runes. In this fourth pillar of Runology, we will learn about the different spreads and layouts you can use in your readings. These spreads and layouts help us determine exactly what these powerful symbols are trying to tell us about our question. When interpreting runes, we look at the meaning of the runic symbol itself (depending on whether it's upright, in opposition, or merkstave) and how it is connected to other runes in the reading. It is this second point that spreads and layouts help us with. Let us get going with the next part of our journey into the world of Runology by learning about the different structures you can use to gain the clearest, most detailed answer from the runes you can.

7

Layouts and Spreads List

When using the runes for divination, it is important to note which runes are present and where they fall in the casting. The sequence in which the runes fall forms a pattern known as a *'spread.'* A spread helps to determine the significance and way to interpret a rune in your reading. For example, your first rune in a reading could represent the past, the second an obstacle, and the third your present situation. Spreads range from two runes to including the full 24 runes of the futhark. All the spreads and layouts we use to *'map'* out the answer we seek are modern inventions. This is because we know precious little about the divination rituals of the ancient people. As such, making the spread you use your own is fun. Some people use the same spread every time they consult their runes, while others like to mix and max depending on the setting, surrounding circumstances, or information sought.

There are many different ways to structure your rune casting. As with whether to use the Elder Futhark, Younger Futhark, or Anglo-Saxon futhorc for your rune set, the choice 0f how to structure your readings is up to you. The previous chapter covered a basic way to begin casting and reading runes. In this one, we will dive in deep, looking at the different kinds of spreads and layouts you can use to enhance and advance your ability to interpret what these symbols of the cosmos are trying to tell you about your question. The more detailed or specific you want your answer, the more complex your spread or layout will be. This is so that more runes are included in the reading.

In this chapter, we are going to cover a wide variety of different layouts and spreads. We will review the simple or smaller layouts or spreads to use for more general questions and those designed for precise, guided answers.

Runic Layouts and Spreads

What is the difference between a layout and a spread? Simply put, a layout was created specifically for rune casting. On the other hand, a spread refers to tarot card spreads adapted for rune readings. While some prefer to keep it traditional and only use layouts for their castings, others feel more connected with the structure of a certain spread. Most people use the terms layout and spread interchangeably in a rune casting. What matters more than this is choosing a layout or spread that best fits your question and your desired answer's details. Let us go through the main layouts and spreads for you to choose from when casting runes.

Single-Rune Layout

The single-rune layout is the simplest way to cast runes, as it involves drawing only one tile. You can draw this single rune from your rune pouch or cast the runes on your casting cloth before, eyes to the sky, picking one. This layout gets a general feeling toward your question rather than specific information. It is also used if you are seeking a quick bit of insight into the main driving force of a certain situation.

Three-Rune Layout

A three-rune layout, also known as the 'past, present, future' layout, is a great way to track the effects or progress of something over time. This layout allows you to structure your casting using time.

If you cast your runes out or draw them from your pouch, ask your question and pick the first tile. This represents the past and the influences and circumstances related to the question. Place this tile on the left and interpret its meaning. Then, ask your question again and draw the next tile. This represents the present and those factors currently affecting your question. Place this tile in the middle in front of you. Ask your question and draw the third tile. This represents the future and is your question's outcome or result.

Fork Spread

Another pattern of the three runes is the fork spread. Like a fork in the road, this spread is used to gain insights when making an important decision or during a great change in your life.

The first tile represents the first possible outcome of your question and is placed on the left. It can also mean one of two choices that you have to make. The second tile is placed right of the center and is the other possible choice or outcome. The final rune is located south of the center (closest to you) and is your question's determining factor or outcome.

Relationship Spread

If you seek insights into what certain people mean to you, this is the layout to use. A relationship spread is a three-rune cast that shows what role people play in our lives. It can also be used to determine what role people play in the lives of others. For example, if you are trying to figure out what your spouse's overly friendly colleague means to them. This layout can also help you to determine the direction of the relationship between people.

Draw the first tile and put it left of center on your casting cloth. This rune is the energy that you are sending out toward this relationship. Draw your next tile and place it next to the first. This rune is the energy your partner puts out regarding the relationship. Finally, draw the third tile and place it above the previous two, connecting them. This rune represents the health and purpose of the relationship.

Four Direction Layout

Norse mythology tells tales of four mighty dvärgar (dwarves) charged with holding up the very sky itself. The dwarves stood in four cardinal directions: *Norðri in the North, Suðri in the South, Austri in the East, and Vestri in the West.*

The first tile of a four-direction layout is Norðri (North). Representing the past, Norðri covers past influences and desires that have led to your present situation. The next tile is Vestri (West), which symbolizes the present situation. A rune in this position gives insights into your current path and the influences you are presently under. The third tile is Austri (East), which deals with the veiled future. It is veiled because a rune in this position only speaks of possible future influences or obstacles that should be watched out for. Finally, we end the four-direction layout with Suðri (South). A rune cast in Suðri represents the possible outcome from the reading. In other words, what could result from you creating a new future using the insights gained from this casting.

Remember, though, that rune casting is not a predictor of the future. It merely offers insights to help and guide you to a desired outcome.

Diamond Spread

The diamond spread uses the same shape as the four-direction layout but with a different order for laying the runes and a different meaning for each position. This is the spread used to divine the forces active and at work in a certain situation or to reveal a hidden conflict or obstacle in your way.

The first tile in this layout is placed south of the center. This rune symbolizes the foundational level of your question and the basic influences acting on it. The next tile goes left of center and tells of one force acting for or against your question. The third rune is placed right of center and represents another force acting for or against the reason for the casting. Finally, the fourth rune is placed north of the center and is the outcome of the casting.

Elemental Spread

Another four-rune reading that forms the same shape as the four-direction layout and diamond spread is the elemental spread. This spread draws on the power of the elements and the forces and qualities they embody. This makes it an excellent option for those who prefer to draw on elemental forces rather than invoke the gods in their casts.

The first tile is placed north of the center and represents Earth. A rune in this position is the lesson you must learn in the physical world. Place the next tile right of the center. This is the air rune, and it represents lessons to learn in the world within your head, your mind. The next element is fire, placed south of the center. These are lessons you need to know in spirit. Finally, the left-center is the water element, representing lessons to learn emotionally.

Five-Rune Cross

The following layout to use in your readings is the five-rune cross. This layout resembles the four-direction layout we covered above, with an extra rune in the middle. While the pattern may be similar, the meaning of each position is very different.

Place the first tile closest to you at the bottom of the cross. This rune will represent the base things influencing your question. The next tile is placed left of center and signifies any obstacles to your question that must be overcome. The third rune is placed at the top of the cross and represents factors that could prove beneficial to answering your question or solving your problem. The right of the cross is the fourth tile, showing a possible outcome to your question. Finally, the fifth rune goes in the middle and symbolizes elements that may influence the outcome in the future.

Medicine Wheel Spread

If you seek a solution to a problem but do not know what course of action to take, then the medicine wheel spread is the layout. This is a five-rune cast with the same pattern as the five-rune cross. The meaning of each position, however, is quite different.

Begin by placing the first tile left of the center. This represents past influences or the origins of the problem. Place the next tile right of the center. This position covers any influences presently affecting your problem. The third tile goes south of the center, closest to you, and shows how the energy of the problem and its solution changes or will change. After that, place your next tile north of the center, symbolizing the problem or challenge itself. Finally, draw the fifth tile and put it in the center to complete the pattern. This rune represents what you should do or the power you need to call on, to solve the problem.

Odin's Layout

Another five-rune cast, Odin's layout, is a more advanced form of the three-rune layout we looked at earlier. Like with its simpler form, Odin's layout is used to gain insights about a particular issue's past, present, and future.

Draw your first tile and place it on the far left of your casting cloth. This position represents the distant past. Your second tile goes next to this one, still left of center, and signifies the recent past. Place the third tile north of the center. This is the present. The last two tiles are placed on the right, with the near future nearest to the center and the distant future next to it on the far side of the pattern.

Grid of Nine

In the Grid of Nine, there are three columns with three runes in each of them. The numbering, however, is not as you would expect it to be. In this layout, you cast out the runes, ask your question, and then pick up nine tiles, selecting them all before interpreting them. The runes are placed in the following order:

$$4\ 9\ 2$$
$$3\ 5\ 7$$
$$8\ 1\ 6$$

When reading the runes using this layout, begin with the lowest line first. This line outlines past influences affecting the subject matter of your question. Start with the eighth rune, which represents hidden past influences to your question. Rune one is next, which shows the basic influences from the past. The final one for the first row is rune six. This tile deals with how you, as the rune caster, feel about these past influences.

Next is the middle row, which is about forces acting on your question. First up in the middle row is the third tile you cast. Like the eighth rune below it in the column, this tile represents hidden influences, but this time those acting on your question in the present. After that, in the middle of the pattern is the fifth rune, which shows the present situation. Last in the middle row is the seventh rune. This is your attitude toward the current state of things related to your question.

The top row covers the outcome of the question you asked. It starts with the fourth tile drawn, which once again represents hidden influences, but this time those related to any obstacles or possible hindrances to the question's positive outcome. Next is the ninth rune, which deals with the best outcome to the subject matter of your question. The final rune in the set is the second tile drawn and signifies your attitude or response to the result of the casting. An interesting note about the Grid of Nine layout is that every row, column, or diagonal line adds up to 15.

Celtic Cross Spread

The Celtic Cross involves a more advanced pattern to use for your readings. When used for a Tarot reading, the first card in this spread is chosen to represent the questioner. For rune casting, you can select a rune that has meaning to you or the person asking the question (if you are doing a reading for someone else). You could also draw this rune randomly from your rune pouch. Either way, this rune will represent the energy of the casting. Draw the symbol on a piece of paper to remember it, and then place the tile back in your pouch so that it can appear in your reading. Concentrate on this rune and how it relates to the clarity or information you seek as you progress through this 10-rune spread.

With your guiding rune chosen and made the focus of the reading, you are now ready to begin. Cast out the runes or draw them one at a time from your pouch. Place the first tile in the center. This rune symbolizes the current situation regarding your question. Draw your second tile and place it on the first rune (if possible). This rune represents the forces that could oppose or be an obstacle to the question. Place the third tile south, in-between you and the first and second runes in the pattern. The third rune tells the hidden or underlying factors influencing the subject matter of your question. The fourth one is placed to the left of the first and second and deals with past influences or those in the process of ending. The fifth is placed in the north, above one and two. This indicates anything that may influence the answer you seek in the future, specifically the medium- to long-term. The sixth tile in the pattern is placed to the right of the first two and shows any influences shortly.

The following four tiles are placed in a column to the left of the sixth, beginning with seven at the bottom and ending with ten at the top. The seventh tile denotes your fears or trepidations toward the question, while the eighth signifies the influences from friends and family. The ninth tile expresses your hopes and beliefs, while the tenth is the outcome of your question.

Celestial Spread

A celestial spread represents a year, beginning with whatever month you are presently in. This is a great layout if you want a month-by-month feel for your question or are looking for an overview of the upcoming year. A celestial spread consists of 13 runes, with the 13th representing the main influence of the year as a whole rather than for a particular month.

The first rune represents the month you are in when you ask your question. Place this rune right of the center and write down its meaning and your interpretation. Then, draw your next tile and place it south of the center. The third rune goes on the left, and the fourth goes north of the center. The fifth tile is placed next to the first on the right, and the pattern continues this way, ending with rune 12 north of the center. As mentioned above, the 13th rune represents the year's primary influence. This tile is placed in the center, completing the pattern.

Pillar 5
Reading

With your question asked, tiles cast, and runes placed in the spread or layout of your choice, there is only one thing left to do—interpret the reading. Welcome, divine rune caster, to the final pillar of runology! Reading runes is not a science but an art. The answer to your question is not going to come in some formulaic or precise manner that automatically solves your problem. However, it will provide insights that help guide your thoughts and consider things from a different (divine) perspective. Reading runes is the culmination of everything we have covered in this book so far and is why you set out on this magical journey to become a rune caster in the first place. Let us look at how to put the runes to work in guiding you to a better tomorrow.

8

Interpreting Runes

While casting runes is pretty simple, interpreting them can be quite tricky. This is because the runes do not give you a straightforward answer but provide insights that help you think through your problems. In this way, the runes guide us, hinting at a solution provided by the unseen powers of the universe and interpreted by the caster. Your intuition and gut feelings play an essential part in reading runes. As we saw in earlier chapters, each rune has a variety of meanings and several different ways that they can be interpreted. The purpose you give each rune needs to consider its inherent meaning, the context of your question, surrounding circumstances, and the other runes in the read. Also, if you are using a layout or a spread, then the position of the rune in the pattern also needs to be considered.

In this chapter, we will go over some final tips for you to use when interpreting the runes of your cast. We will review how to cast and interpret your runes and end by providing you with a summary of the runes and their meanings. Let us get this final part of your runic journey underway!

Casting and Interpreting Runes

When reading runes, focus on how they relate to your life and the question you are asking. Do not focus solely on the rune itself, but always think about how the cosmos' powerful principles and forces represent themselves in your lived experience. For example, Fehu merkstave could signify losses through gambling, or it could be interpreted as losing one's wealth of spirit or self-esteem.

This section summarizes the runic symbols, sounds, and meanings that we looked at in Pillar 2: Runic Scripts. Use this summary when reading the runes to help you interpret them quickly and efficiently. This will help to ensure you do not lose the flow of the moment during a casting. The more you cast and interpret runes, the more familiar you will get with them. Initially, it will require much checking up on the rune meanings. It will also take time to consider how that meaning fits in with your question and into the position it falls in the pattern.

This summary will focus on the 24 runes found in the Elder Futhark. This is because these are the runes usually used for casting runes. We will, however, also go through the Younger Futhark and Anglo-Saxon futhorc equivalents to these runes. Remember that the meanings of these powerful symbols of cosmic forces and universal principles are not set in stone. They should always be considered in the light of your own lived experience. The following summary merely serves as a guide to help you understand what the runes are trying to tell you in that casting.

Freyr/Freyja's Ætt

Fehu	
Rune	ᚠ
Meaning	Wealth (cattle)
Symbolizes	Possessions and values
Sound	/f/ , /v/
Younger Futhark	Fé (ᚠ)
Anglo-Saxon futhorc	Feoh (ᚠ)
Upright	Hope, abundance, and success
Merkstave	Loss of something you value

Ūruz	
Rune	ᚢ
Meaning	Aurochs (wild ox)
Symbolizes	Physical strength and untamed potential
Sound	/u/
Younger Futhark	Úr (ᚢ) 'rain'
Anglo-Saxon futhorc	Ur (ᚢ)
Upright	Shaping of power; positive changes
Merkstave	Misdirected efforts or ignorant actions

Thurisaz	
Rune	þ
Meaning	Giant

The 5 Pillars of Runes

Symbolizes	Connection and opposition; brute strength
Sound	/þ/ (/th/)
Younger Futhark	Þhurs (þ)
Anglo-Saxon futhorc	Þorn (Þ) 'thorn'
Upright	Reactive or directed force; vitality and instinct-based willpower
Merkstave	Danger, betrayal, malice

Ansuz	
Rune	ᚠ
Meaning	God (Odin)
Symbolizes	Insight and communication with your higher self
Sound	/a/
Younger Futhark	Óss (ᚯ)
Anglo-Saxon futhorc	Ōs (ᚠ) 'god'; Āc (ᚠ) 'oak'; Æsc (ᚠ) 'ash'
Upright	Insight, inspiration, wisdom, harmony
Merkstave	Misunderstanding, manipulation, delusion

Raidho	
Rune	ᚱ
Meaning	Ride
Symbolizes	Travel, movement, the journey of life

Sound	/r/
Younger Futhark	Reið (ᚱ)
Anglo-Saxon futhorc	Rād (ᚱ)
Upright	Personal evolution; a sign you are on the right path
Merkstave	Disruption or disconnection; an omen of death

Kaunan	
Rune	ᚲ
Meaning	ulcer
Symbolizes	Wisdom or enlightenment
Sound	/k/
Younger Futhark	Kaun (ᚴ)
Anglo-Saxon futhorc	Cēn/Kenaz (ᚳ) 'torch'
Upright	Revelation, positive transformation, revitalized energy
Merkstave	Sickness, stagnation, suffering; arrogance, ignorance, elitism

Gebo	
Rune	X
Meaning	gift
Symbolizes	The balance between give and take
Sound	/g/
Younger Futhark	
Anglo-Saxon futhorc	Gyfu (X)

Upright	Rewards for sacrifices made, clarity of vision, divine blessing
In opposition	Loneliness, greed, overdependence; over self-sacrificing, bribery

Wunjo	
Rune	ᚹ
Meaning	Joy or bliss
Symbolizes	Hope, harmony, love, togetherness
Sound	/w/; /v/
Younger Futhark	
Anglo-Saxon futhorc	Wynn (ᚹ)
Upright	Comfort, contentment, fellowship; glory and spiritual rewards
Merkstave	Alienation or possession; frenzy or berserker's rage

Heimdall's Ætt

Hagalaz	
Rune	H
Meaning	Hail
Symbolizes	Sudden change; creative and destructive forces
Sound	/h/
Younger Futhark	Hagall (✱)
Anglo-Saxon futhorc	Hægl (ᚻ)

Upright	Resilience, tempering, inner strength and willpower; growth and balance
In opposition	Powerlessness, suffering, impending disaster

Naudiz	
Rune	ᚾ
Meaning	Need or constraint
Symbolizes	Necessity and difficulty; restrictions required to build inner strength
Sound	/n/
Younger Futhark	Nauðr (ᚾ)
Anglo-Saxon futhorc	Nȳd (ᚾ)
Upright	Endurance, determination, restraint, patience; coming to terms with orlog
Merkstave	Restriction or loss of freedom; want or unmet emotional needs

Isaz	
Rune	ᛁ
Meaning	ice
Symbolizes	Self-control; stillness and fortitude of mind
Sound	/i/
Younger Futhark	Íss (ᛁ)
Anglo-Saxon futhorc	Īs (ᛁ)
Upright	Overcoming challenges; developing self-awareness and clarity

In opposition	Egocentricity, loss of control, over-indulgence in sensory pleasures; betrayal or treachery

Jēran	
Rune	ᚼ
Meaning	Year or harvest
Symbolizes	Reward for hard work and positive actions
Sound	/j/
Younger Futhark	Ár (ᛏ)
Anglo-Saxon futhorc	Gēr (ᚼ)
Upright	Positive results for earlier efforts, peace, prosperity; success and happiness
In opposition	Poor timing or an unexpected setback; reversal of luck and fortune

Eihwaz	
Rune	ᛇ
Meaning	Yew tree; Yggdrasil
Symbolizes	Life, death, and renewal
Sound	/y/
Younger Futhark	
Anglo-Saxon futhorc	Ēoh (ᛇ)
Upright	Enlightenment, protection, are on the right path to achieving your goals
Merkstave	Distraction or dissatisfaction; weakness or confusion

Perthro	
Rune	⌐
Meaning	Lot cup
Symbolizes	Orlog, fate, and the game of life
Sound	/p/
Younger Futhark	
Anglo-Saxon futhorc	Peorð (⌐)
Upright	Good luck and success; determining your own destiny
Merkstave	Stagnation or unhappiness; circumstances beyond your control

Algiz	
Rune	Y
Meaning	Elk or protection
Symbolizes	Spiritual connection with the divine
Sound	/z/
Younger Futhark	Yr (ᛣ) 'yew'
Anglo-Saxon futhorc	Eolh (Y)
Upright	Divine protection, spiritual awakening, connection with your higher self
Merkstave	Weakening of your divine link or repelling; impending danger if things do not change

Sowilō	
Rune	ᛋ
Meaning	Sun

Symbolizes	Success, accomplishment, honor
Sound	/s/
Younger Futhark	Sól (ᛋ)
Anglo-Saxon futhorc	Sigel (ᛋ)
Upright	Guidance and hope; positive change and achieving victory
Merkstave	Disconnection, false success, bad advice; losing sight of goals and purpose

Týr's Ætt

Tiwaz	
Rune	↑
Meaning	Týr
Symbolizes	Honor, justice, leadership
Sound	/t/
Younger Futhark	Týr (↑)
Anglo-Saxon futhorc	Tīr (↑)
Upright	Justice, victory, coming to terms with the self-sacrifice required to succeed
Merkstave	Over-analyzing, injustice, failure; diminishing of purpose and passion

Berkanen	
Rune	ᛒ
Meaning	Birch tree
Symbolizes	Fertility, cycle of life and death, new growth, rebirth

Sound	/b/
Younger Futhark	Björk (ᛒ)
Anglo-Saxon futhorc	Beorc (ᛒ)
Upright	Renewal, positive change, the beginning of something new
In opposition	Anxiety, domestic problems, blurred vision; forces conspiring against you

Ehwaz	
Rune	ᛖ
Meaning	Horse
Symbolizes	Movement and progress
Sound	/e/
Younger Futhark	
Anglo-Saxon futhorc	Eh (ᛖ)
Upright	Harmony, steady progress, loyalty
Merkstave	Disharmony, indecisiveness, betrayal

Mannaz	
Rune	ᛗ
Meaning	Man or Humankind
Symbolizes	Intelligence, planning, heightened awareness
Sound	/m/
Younger Futhark	Maðr (ᛘ)
Anglo-Saxon futhorc	Mann (ᛗ)

Upright	Self-actualization, divine influence, creativity
Merkstave	Mortality, destructive emotions, shortcomings of humankind

Laguz	
Rune	ᛚ
Meaning	Lake or water
Symbolizes	Life energy, collective memory, purification
Sound	/l/
Younger Futhark	Lögr (ᛚ)
Anglo-Saxon futhorc	Lagu (ᛚ)
Upright	Imagination, dreams, balance, growth; on-track to achieving your goals
Merkstave	Tumult, confusion, poor judgment; stuck in a downward spiral

Inguz	
Rune	ᛜ
Meaning	Ing (Freyr)
Symbolizes	Male fertility, internal growth, creation
Sound	/ŋ/
Younger Futhark	
Anglo-Saxon futhorc	Ing (ᛝ)
Upright	Self-improvement, gestation, growth

In opposition	Immaturity, frivolity, effort without gain

Dagaz	
Rune	ᛞ
Meaning	Day
Symbolizes	Awakening or enlightenment
Sound	/d/
Younger Futhark	
Anglo-Saxon futhorc	Dæg (ᛞ)
Upright	Hope, happiness, certainty; heightened awareness and positivity
In opposition	Lacking vision or hopelessness

Othala	
Rune	ᛟ
Meaning	Heritage or inheritance
Symbolizes	Home, connection with your ancestors, spiritual roots
Sound	/o/
Younger Futhark	
Anglo-Saxon futhorc	Ēðel (ᛟ)
Upright	Prosperity, freedom, safety, spiritual aid
Merkstave	Losing touch with heritage, poverty, mistreatment

Conclusion

Welcome, my freshly initiated runologist, to the end of this book! We have taken quite the learning journey together as we traversed our way through the five pillars of runology. By absorbing the knowledge, techniques, and strategies in this book, you have taken more than a few steps forward on your path toward enlightenment. That is the true glory of runelore; we discover more about ourselves as we learn about these powerful symbols of cosmic forces and universal principles.

Whether you use the Elder Futhark, Younger Futhark, or Anglo-Saxon futhorc for your castings or a spread or a layout, the result is the same. You will gain insights into the hidden workings of the world and guidance on how to deal with any problems or obstacles that arise on your life's journey.

Reading runes requires more feeling than thinking. It is about the energy you bring to the casting, the divine powers you invoke, and the emotions and intuitions you feel as you interpret the tiles. It is not a science, but it often offers insights that no scientific process could provide you with.

Because it is about feelings, you should make rune casting your own. Create your own ritual space for casting runes, using the Hammarsetning to sanctify the space. Select a material for your rune tiles that resonates most with your psyche and design your casting cloth, rune pouch, and stol in a way that best captures what these ancient magical symbols mean to you. Finally, choose mearmots (personal talismans) that get you in the right frame of mind and emotional state for reading and interpreting runes, using a spread or layout that best maps out the answer you seek.

It is as simple as that! You are ready to use the runes to improve your life and those around you. Get in touch with your inner Viking and call on the wisdom of the runes to enhance your life's story. The world is full of mystery and wonder. Learn how to read these signs and tap into the wisdom of the divine through the power of the runes.

References List

A Little Sparkle of Joy. (2022). *The 24 Runes Meanings and How to Access Their Magic*. Www.alittlesparkofjoy.com. https://www.alittlesparkofjoy.com/runes/

Bellows, H. A. (2007). *The poetic Edda : the heroic poems*. Dover Publications.

Beltane, C. (2021a). *Anglo-Saxon and Frisian Rune*. Witches of the Craft®. https://witchesofthecraft.com/tag/anglo-saxon-and-frisian-rune/

Beltane, C. (2021b). *Norse Runes: Viking Runes, Norse Symbols & Much More to Know!* Witches of the Craft®. https://witchesofthecraft.com/2021/11/03/norse-runes-viking-runes-norse-symbols-much-more-to-know/

Caro, T. (2020). *What Does the Othala Rune Mean? [Upright, Reversed & Uses]*. Magickalspot.com. https://magickalspot.com/othala-rune/

Connolly, L. (2021). *The Younger Futhark*. The Spells8 Forum. https://forum.spells8.com/t/the-younger-futhark/10365

Forefathers Art. (2019a). *Anglo-Saxon Runes - Futhorc of the Anglo-Saxons*. Forefathers-Art.com. https://forefathers-art.com/anglo-saxon-runes-futhorc-of-the-anglo-saxons

Forefathers Art. (2019b). *Younger Futhark - The Meanings of the Runes*. Forefathers-Art.com. https://forefathers-art.com/younger-futhark-the-meanings-of-the-runes

Gronitz, D. (2010). *Younger Futhork – Rune Meanings*. Www.therunesite.com. http://www.therunesite.com/younger-futhork-rune-meanings/#:~:text=The%20Younger%20Futhork%20consists%20of%2016%20runes%20and

Guido. (2022). *Tyr's Ætt*. Mind Unfolded. https://sites.google.com/site/mindunfolded/chapter-6/tyr-s-aett-1

Harris, J. (2022). *Runemarks: Using Runes | Joanne Harris*. Joanneharris.co.uk. http://www.joanne-harris.co.uk/books/runemarks/runemarks-using-runes/

Hill, B. (2019). *Futhark: Mysterious Ancient Runic Alphabet of Northern Europe*. Ancient Origins Reconstructing the Story of Humanity's Past. https://www.ancient-origins.net/artifacts-ancient-writings/futhark-mysterious-ancient-runic-alphabet-northern-europe-003250

Hubbard, E., Tuit, L., & Lewis, D. (2022). *Introduction to Runes*. Witchschool.com. https://witchschool.com/lesson_detail/539?page=1

Khan, M. (2019a). *Calc the Cup: Northumbrian Runes*. Heathen at Heart. https://www.patheos.com/blogs/heathenatheart/2019/06/calc-the-cup/

Khan, M. (2019b). *Cweorth: Northumbrian Runes*. Heathen at Heart. https://www.patheos.com/blogs/heathenatheart/2019/07/cweorth-northumbrian-runes/

Khan, M. (2019c). *Gar the Spear: Northumbrian Runes*. Heathen at Heart. https://www.patheos.com/blogs/heathenat-heart/2019/07/gar-the-spear-northumbrian-runes/

Leeming, D. (2005). Poetic Edda. In The Oxford Companion to World Mythology. : Oxford University Press. Retrieved 2 Dec. 2022, from https://www.oxfordreference.com/view/10.1093/acref/9780195156690.001.0001/acref-9780195156690-e-1274.

Linton, M. (2013). *All About Runes A Book of Runes A Wikipedia Compilation*. http://www.1066.co.nz/Mosaic%20DVD/library/runes/all%20about%20runes.pdf#page=96

Linton, M. A. (2013). *All about Runes A Book of Runes*. http://www.1066.co.nz/Mosaic%20DVD/library/runes/all%20about%20runes.pdf#page=96

Mart, L. (2014). *Divination 1: Question 5 (Rune Meanings)*. Little Druid on the Prairie. https://prairiedruid.com/2014/06/06/divination-1-question-5-rune-meanings/

McCoy, D. (2012a). *Runes*. Norse Mythology for Smart People. https://norse-mythology.org/runes/

McCoy, D. (2012b). *Runic Philosophy and Magic - Norse Mythology for Smart People*. Norse Mythology for Smart People. https://norse-mythology.org/runes/runic-philosophy-and-magic/

McCoy, D. (2012c). *The Binding of Fenrir*. Norse Mythology for Smart People. https://norse-mythology.org/tales/the-binding-of-fenrir/

Modern Norse Heathen. (2017). *A Beginner's Guide to Rune Casting*. Modern Norse Heathen. https://modernnorseheathen.wordpress.com/2017/09/13/a-beginners-guide-to-rune-casting/

Newcombe, R. (2019). *Rune Guide - An Introduction to using the Runes*. Holistic Shop. https://www.holisticshop.co.uk/articles/guide-runes

Omniglot. (2019). *Anglo-Saxon runes (Futhorc)*. https://www.omniglot.com/writing/futhorc.htm

Rhys, D. (2021). *Algiz Rune – History and Meaning*. Symbol Sage. https://symbolsage.com/algiz-rune-symbol-meaning/

RODNAE Productions. (2021). Top View of Astrology Items [Online Image]. In *Pexels*.

Rune Secrets. (2020). *How to Interpret the Runes*. Rune Secrets. https://runesecrets.com/rune-lore/how-to-interpret-the-runes

Saul, F. (2017). *Elder Futhark*. Auntyflo.com. https://www.auntyflo.com/spiritual-meaning/elder-futhark

Sawyer, A. (2021). *Elder Futhark Runes — Meanings And Rune Casting Basics*. YourTango. https://www.yourtango.com/2018316703/how-to-read-cast-interpret-rune-casting-astrology-zodiac-horoscope

Starfire, L. (2018). *The Three Aettirs of the Elder Futhark Runes*. Witches of the Craft®. https://witchesofthecraft.com/2018/09/12/the-three-aettirs-of-the-elder-futhark-runes/

Symbolikon. (2023). *Thurisaz - Norse Runes symbol - Symbolikon Worldwide Symbols*. Symbolikon.com. https://symbolikon.com/downloads/thurisaz-norse-runes/#:~:text=Thurisaz%20is%20a%20protective%20rune

Taylor, K. E. (2020). *Futhorc: The Anglo-Saxon Runes & Runology*. Druidry. https://druidry.org/resources/futhorc-the-anglo-saxon-runes-runology

The English Companions. (2021). *About the Anglo-Saxon Futhorc.* https://www.tha-engliscan-gesithas.org.uk/written-and-spoken-old-english/old-english-alphabet-2/about-the-anglo-saxon-futhorc/

The Pagan Grimoire. (2022). *Your Guide to the 24 Elder Futhark Runes and Their Meanings.* The Pagan Grimoire. https://www.pagangrimoire.com/elder-futhark-rune-meanings/

The Rune Site. (2010, September 27). *Northumbrian Runes – Rune Meanings.* Www.therunesite.com. http://www.therunesite.com/northumbrian-runes-rune-meanings/

The Viking Rune. (2008). *Younger Futhark Runes: The Rune Set Used by Norse Vikings.* Vikingrune.com. https://www.vikingrune.com/2008/11/younger-futhark-runes/

Two Wander. (2020). *Rune Meanings and How to Use Rune Stones for Divination.* Two Wander. https://www.twowander.com/blog/rune-meanings-how-to-use-runestones-for-divination

Tyler, D. (2015). *Your Guide to Rune Divination.* Rune Divination. https://runedivination.com/your-guide-to-rune-divination/

Tyler, D. (2019). *Casting Runes.* Rune Divination. https://runedivination.com/casting-runes/

Tyriel. (2008a). *Algiz - Rune Meaning.* Rune Secrets. https://runesecrets.com/rune-meanings/algiz

Tyriel. (2008b). *Ansuz - Rune Meaning.* Rune Secrets. https://runesecrets.com/rune-meanings/ansuz

Tyriel. (2008c). *Berkano - Rune Meaning.* Rune Secrets. https://runesecrets.com/rune-meanings/berkano

Tyriel. (2008d). *Dagaz - Rune Meaning*. Rune Secrets. https://runesecrets.com/rune-meanings/dagaz

Tyriel. (2008e). *Ehwaz - Rune Meaning*. Rune Secrets. https://runesecrets.com/rune-meanings/ehwaz

Tyriel. (2008f). *Fehu - Rune Meaning*. Rune Secrets. https://runesecrets.com/

Tyriel. (2008g). *Gebo - Rune Meaning*. Rune Secrets. https://runesecrets.com/rune-meanings/gebo

Tyriel. (2008h). *Hagalaz - Rune Meaning*. Rune Secrets. https://runesecrets.com/rune-meanings/hagalaz

Tyriel. (2008i). *Ihwaz or Eihwaz - Rune Meaning*. Rune Secrets. https://runesecrets.com/rune-meanings/ihwaz-eihwaz

Tyriel. (2008j). *Inguz - Rune Meaning*. Rune Secrets. https://runesecrets.com/rune-meanings/inguz

Tyriel. (2008k). *Isa - Rune Meaning*. Rune Secrets. https://runesecrets.com/rune-meanings/isa

Tyriel. (2008l). *Jera - Rune Meaning*. Rune Secrets. https://runesecrets.com/rune-meanings/jera

Tyriel. (2008m). *Kenaz - Rune Meaning*. Rune Secrets. https://runesecrets.com/rune-meanings/kenaz

Tyriel. (2008n). *Laguz - Rune Meaning*. Rune Secrets. https://runesecrets.com/rune-meanings/laguz

Tyriel. (2008o). *Mannaz - Rune Meaning*. Rune Secrets. https://runesecrets.com/rune-meanings/mannaz

Tyriel. (2008p). *Nauthiz - Rune Meaning*. Rune Secrets. https://runesecrets.com/rune-meanings/nauthiz

Tyriel. (2008q). *Othala - Rune Meaning*. Rune Secrets. https://runesecrets.com/rune-meanings/othala

Tyriel. (2008r). *Perthro - Rune Meaning*. Rune Secrets. https://runesecrets.com/rune-meanings/perthro

Tyriel. (2008s). *Raidho - Rune Meaning*. Rune Secrets. https://runesecrets.com/rune-meanings/raidho

Tyriel. (2008t). *Sowilo - Rune Meaning*. Rune Secrets. https://runesecrets.com/rune-meanings/sowilo

Tyriel. (2008u). *Thurisaz - Rune Meaning*. Rune Secrets. https://runesecrets.com/rune-meanings/thurisaz

Tyriel. (2008v). *Tiwaz - Rune Meaning*. Rune Secrets. https://runesecrets.com/rune-meanings/tiwaz

Tyriel. (2008w). *Uruz - Rune Meaning*. Rune Secrets. https://runesecrets.com/rune-meanings/uruz

Tyriel. (2008x). *Wunjo - Rune Meaning*. Rune Secrets. https://runesecrets.com/rune-meanings/wunjo

van der Hoeven, J. (2020). *The Runes:* Ōs. Down the Forest Path. https://downtheforestpath.com/2020/11/26/the-runes-os/

van der Hoeven, J. (2022). *The Runes: Rād*. Down the Forest Path. https://downtheforestpath.com/tag/runes/#:~:text=The%20fifth%20rune%2C%20R%C4%81d%20or

Viking Style. (2020). *Viking Rune Meanings*. Viking Style. https://viking.style/viking-rune-meanings/

Wigington, P. (2020). *What Is Rune Casting? Origins and Techniques*. Learn Religions. https://www.learnreligions.com/rune-casting-4783609

Williamson, J. (2022). *All you need to know about the Elder Futhark, the oldest form of runic alphabets*. The Viking Herald. https://thevikingherald.com/article/all-you-need-to-know-about-the-elder-futhark-the-oldest-form-of-runic-alphabets/294

Made in the USA
Middletown, DE
27 January 2024